A Guide
to the
Study
of BASIC
MEDICAL MYCOLOGY

Kee Peng Ng, Tuck Soon Soo-Hoo & Shiang Ling Na

ISBN
978-1-4828-2412-4 (sc)
978-1-4828-2413-1 (e)

To order additional copies of this book, contact
Toll Free 800 101 2657 (Singapore)
Toll Free 1 800 81 7340 (Malaysia)
orders.singapore@partridgepublishing.com

www.partridgepublishing.com/singapore

09/10/2014

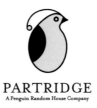

PARTRIDGE
A Penguin Random House Company

Contents

Preface

Mycotic diseases are gaining importance as a result of the increase in the incidence of opportunistic fungal infections among immunocompromised patients. The identification of fungi isolated from clinical material has posed a variety of problems to many laboratories due to lack of expertise and experience, especially in the identification of recently emerged rare fungi that had not been previously reported.

Mycology is a small component of microbiology as taught in the undergraduate medical course. The exposure of most medical students to basic mycology is limited to a few medically important fungal species such as *Candida, Cryptococcus, Aspergillus,* and the dermatophytes. However many of the recently recognized fungal pathogens, such as the dematiaceous fungi, are seldom included in the teaching modules. This will handicap young medical graduates when confronted with the ever increasing number of fungal pathogens.

This illustrated guide is meant to provide, as comprehensively as possible, the basic characteristics of fungi frequently isolated from clinical specimens. All the fungi illustrated in this manual are isolated from clinical material obtained in the Mycology Laboratory, Department of Medical Microbiology, Faculty of Medicine, University of Malaya.

The macro- and microscopic features of each fungus are graphically and pictorially presented, and it is hoped that this study guide will be useful to students in their study of clinically important fungi.

Section 1. Introduction to Basic Mycology

Fungi include two diverse forms: moulds and yeasts.

A yeast colony is usually single, round, raised, or convex. The colony may be white, red, or black in colour (Fig. 1A). The vegetative structure of yeast is single, unicellular cells, 4-8 μm in diameter with buddings (Fig. 1B). The yeasts may produce pseudohyphae or true hyphae (Table 1) and reproduce by budding.

A mould colony is fuzzy or cottony in appearance (Fig. 2A). A single growing vegetative structure of mould is known as a hypha or hyphae (more than one hypha). The hyphae can be non-septated (Fig. 2B) or septated and branched (Fig. 2C). The mycelium growing on the surface of the agar medium is called aerial mycelium, and those growing down into the agar are called vegetative mycelium. A mould colony is therefore made up of aerial and vegetative mycelia, which are referred to as thallus (thalli).

Most of the fungi isolated in the clinical laboratory produce only asexual spores. Identification of moulds is made based on the characteristics of the spores and their method of reproduction.

A number of moulds reproduce as yeast-like cells on enriched media when incubated at 37°C or in tissue. The fungi are in mould form on SDA (Sabouraud Dextrose Agar) when incubated at a lower temperature, e.g. 30°C. This phenomenon of changing vegetative structures is called dimorphism. As temperature is a critical factor in the formation of dimorphic characteristic, the phenomenon is also called thermal dimorphism.

Figure 1. Colonial morphology and microscopic appearance of yeast

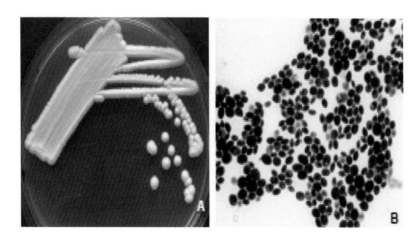

Figure 2. Colonial and microscopic morphology of mould

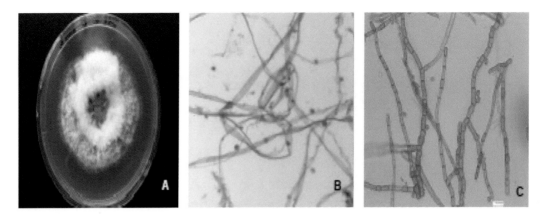

Table 1. The differences between pseudohyphae and hyphae

Pseudohyphae	Hyphae
Growth is by budding process: formation of a new blastoconidium, each with a basal constriction without separation from its parent cell.	Growth is by linear elongation of hyphal apex, with or without septum.
The terminal cell is usually shorter than the preceding cell behind the septum. Wall has invagination at the septum.	The terminal cell is longer than the preceding cells behind the septum. Wall has no invagination at the septum.
The first septum and the side branch are constricted at the point of origin.	The first septum and side branch are not constricted at the point of origin.

Classification of fungi

There are four recognized divisions in the kingdom of fungi: Chytridiomycota, Zygomycota, Ascomycota and Basidiomycota. Members of Chytridiomycota are plant pathogens.

The anamorphic fungi or *fungi imperfecti* (Deuteromycota) refer to groups of fungi not included in these divisions. These fungi only reproduce asexually without a sexual reproductive stage (telemorph). Some of the fungi in the groups that have telemorphs are placed in the Ascomycota or Basidiomycota.

The anamorphic fungi are artificially classified according to the vegetative form of growth and the characteristic production of asexual spores. These fungi are classified into Blastomycetes, Hyphomycetes, and Coelomycetes (Table 2).

The Hyphomycetes produce no fruiting body, and the hyphae are septated. The arrangement and size of conidia depend on the species. Coelomycetes have septate hyphae, and the conidia are produced in fruiting bodies called pycnidia or acervuli. Blastomycetes are yeast-like fungi.

Most of the medically important fungi are within the Blastomycetes, Hyphomycetes and Zygomycetes. The key features listed in Table 3 can be used as a simplified guide to identify the major groups of fungi frequently isolated in a routine clinical mycology laboratory.

Characteristics of fungi

Yeasts

The colonies are single, round, and moist-to-waxy. The cells are predominantly unicellular; they may be spherical, elliptical, or cylindrical. They may be variable in size, ranging from 4-8 µm.

On Cornmeal-Tween 80 agar, many types of yeasts produce pseudohyphae, but a number of yeast-like fungi produce true hyphae.

On a gram stained smear, the yeast cells may be spherical or cylindrical with a predominance of budding cells (Fig. 3A, B). The new cell is abstracted from the mother cell and then enlarged to form a matured cell.

Figure 3. Gram stained smears of yeasts showing budding cells and variability of sizes

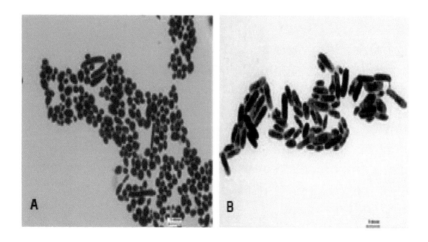

Table 2. Classification of clinically important fungi

Zygomycota
Class: Zygomycetes

       - hyphae are aseptate; mycelium is broad and forms sporangia with nonmotile sporangiospores

       - can produce sexual zygospores

       Order: Mucorales

              Family: *Mucoraceae*

                    Genus: *Rhizopus*

                    Genus: *Mucor*

                    Genus: *Absidia*

              Family: *Cunninghamellaceae*

                    Genus: *Cunninghamella*

              Family: *Syncephalastraceae*

                    Genus: *Syncephalastrum*

       Order: Entomophthorales

              Family: *Basidiobolaceae*

                    Genus: *Basidiobolus*

Ascomycota
Class: Ascomycetes

       - known as true yeasts

       - unicellular forms reproduce asexually by budding or sexually by the formation of ascospores typically with 8 asci

Basidiomycota
Class: Basidiomycetes

       - septate hyphae with clamp connections

       - sexual reproduction by means of basidiospores, typically four, on a basidium

Deuteromycota (*fungi imperfecti*)

       - unicellular or filamentous forms with septate mycelium

       - reproduce asexually by budding. The conidia are borne on conidiophores or in pycnidium or acervulus

       - sexual reproduction absent

Class Hyphomycetes

       - conidia born on conidiophores or directly on hyphae

       - mycelium, conidia and conidiophores may be hyaline or darkly coloured

Class Blastomycetes

       - asexual reproduction by budding

       - yeast-like fungi with or without pseudohyphae or hyphae

       - colonies may be white, red, or black

Class Coelomycetes

       - conidia born in pycnidium or acervulus

Table 3. Important features to identify the medically important fungi

Fungus has no hyphae, consists of abundant budding cells → the colonies are white or red → the colonies are black	Yeasts Black yeasts
Fungus has mycelium → septate with clamp connections → septate, no clamp connections with fruiting bodies containing spores in asci → septate, no clamp connections with fruiting bodies containing loose conidia → septate, no clamp connections, no fruiting bodies	Basidiomycetes Ascomycetes Coelomycetes Hyphomycetes
Fungus has mycelium → aseptate, sporulation abundant	Zygomycetes
Fungi identified only in tissue, not able to grow on routine culture media	*Rhinosporidium seeberi,* *Pneumocystis carinii*

Moulds

The colonies are made up of hyphae and grow by elongation at the tips or by lateral branching, forming a tangled mass of hyphae called mycelium (Fig. 4A, B). The hyphae may become specialized cells that produce conidia called conidiogenous cells.

The conidiophores are morphologically distinct from the vegetative hyphae.

In some fungi, e.g. *Acremonium,* the conidiophores and conidiogenous cells are actually one and the same structures.

In *Aspergillus* or *Penicillium*, conidiogenous cells and conidiophores are two distinctly different structures.

Figure 4. Lactophenol Cotton Blue staining demonstrates nonseptated hyphae (A), septated hyphae and conidiogenous cells (B)

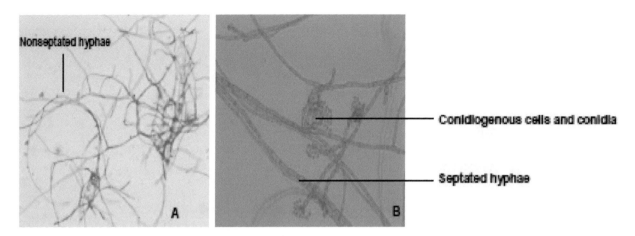

Describing the colonial morphology

All medically important fungi grow on Sabouraud Dextrose Agar (SDA). The description of the morphological characteristics of fungi is normally based on the cultural appearance on SDA incubated at 30°C.

1. Rate of growth: a rapid grower produces characteristic morphology on SDA within five days. A moderate grower produces characteristic morphology between five to ten days, while a slow-growing fungus may take two to three weeks to develop a characteristic morphology.

2. Texture: describing the height of the aerial mycelium (Fig. 5).

   - Yeast-like: colony solid, no production of aerial mycelium (Fig. 5A).
   - Cottony or woolly: fungus produces highly dense aerial mycelium (Fig. 5B).
   - Velvety: colonies produce a low, compact aerial mycelium (Fig. 5C).
   - Granular or powdery: colonies are flat and crumbly with dense conidia production. The granular texture is rough, like granulated sugar; the powdery texture is like flour (Fig. 5D).
   - Labrous or waxy: colonies are smooth, produce no aerial mycelium.

Figure 5. The texture of fungi that grow on SDA

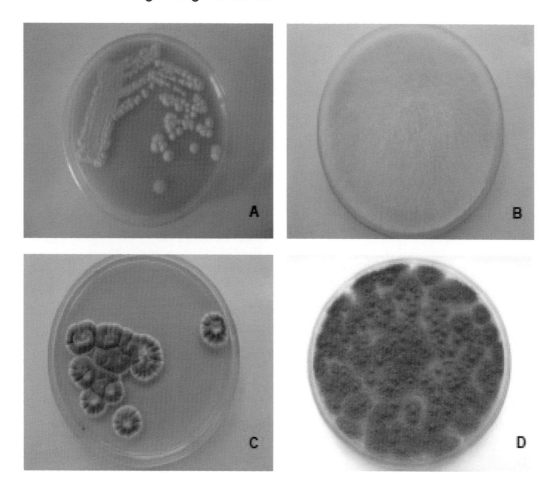

3. Topography: describes the physical appearance of fungal cultures (Fig. 6).

- Flat with radial folds (Fig. 6A).

- Rugose: colonies have deep furrows, irregularly radiating from the centre with entire edge (Fig. 6B).

- Umbonate: colonies possess a button-like central elevation. They may be accompanied by rugose furrows around the button. The edge may be entire or scalloped (Fig. 6C).

- Verrucose: colonies exhibit a wrinkled, convoluted surface (Fig. 6D).

- Cerebriform: colonies exhibit many brain-like folds (Fig. 6E).

Figure 6. The topography of fungi that grow on SDA

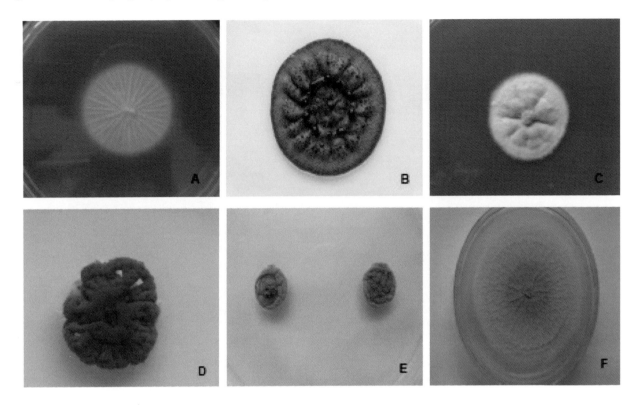

It is important to describe the topographic characteristic of the reverse side of the culture plate like the colour and the presence of radial folds or ridges (Fig. 6F).

4. Colour: the pigmentation of the colony is variable depending on cultural conditions. The pigmentation of the culture is related to the pigmentation of the spores or vegetative hyphae (Fig. 7).

- The colour on the reverse colony is the soluble pigments produced by the fungus diffused into the medium and the original pigmentation of the hyphae.

Figure 7. Colour and soluble pigments produced by fungi

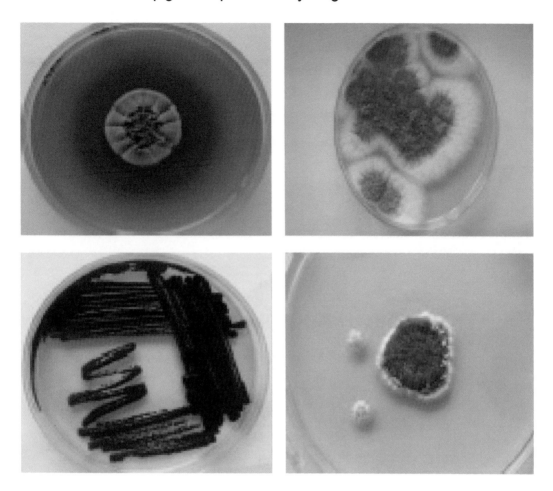

The type of spores

Most clinically important fungi belong to *fungi imperfecti* and produce only asexual spores.

The spores (also called conidia) are produced by segmentation or budding of the tips of the hyphae or from the walls of hyphae. The conidiogenous cell is the hyphal structure that produces conidia.

a. Arthroconidia

- The fragmentation of hypha forms a chain of uniformly sized asexual spores (Fig. 8A).
- These conidia may be randomly arranged (Fig. 8B) in the hyphae or separated by a sterile cell called a disjunctor, e.g. *Geotrichum, Trichosporon, Hendersonula toruloidea, Malbranchea*.

Figure 8. Chain of uniformly and randomly arranged arthroconidia

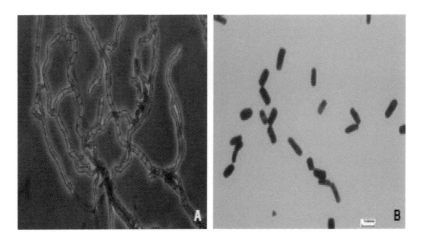

b. Chlamydospores

- They are produced by the cells of pseudohyphae or true hyphae of many filamentous fungi or *Candida* species.

- They are resting spores, thick-walled and heat resistant, and can be terminal (form at the end of hyphae, Ch) (Fig. 9A) or intercalary (form in the hyphae, In) (Fig. 9B).

Figure 9. Chlamydospores produced on Cornmeal-Tween 80 agar

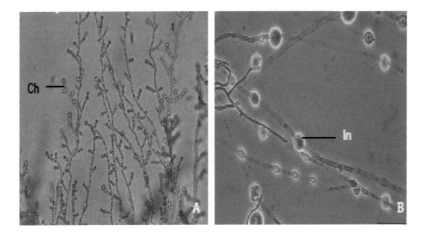

c. Blastospores (Bl)

- These are formed by budding. The young daughter cell is abstracted from the parent cell and then enlarges itself to form a new mature cell (Fig. 10).

Figure 10. Blastospores and pseudomycelium formation on Cornmeal-Tween 80 agar

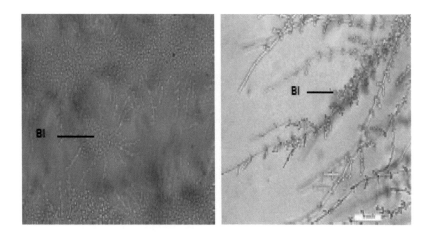

d. Aleuriospores

- These can be sessile or lateral aleuriospores that develop directly on the vegetative mycelium called conidiophore. The phialides produce aleuriospores which can be single-celled (microaleuriospore) or multi-celled (macroaleuriospore).

Figure 11. Aleuriospores and related structures

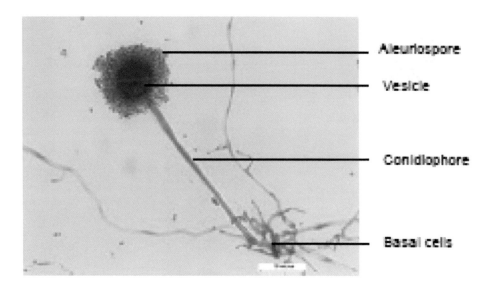

The conidiophore of *Aspergillus* arises from a basal cell on the hypha and enlarges at the end to form a vesicle. Flask-shaped phialides develop over the surface of the vesicle, and conidia are produced successively from the tip of the phialides (Fig. 11). The spores are usually formed in chains. The phialides may be borne directly on the vesicle (uniseriate) (Fig. 12A) or may be borne on prophialides that arise from the vesicle (biseriate) (Fig. 12B).

The terminal portion of conidiophore of *Penicillium* branches into finger-like projections called metulae from which flask-shaped phialides are formed. Conidia (aleuriospores) are abstracted from the tip of the phialides in chains. The conidiophore can be monoverticillate (unbranched), biverticillate, or terverticillate (Fig. 13).

Figure 12. Uniseriate (A) and biseriate (B) arrangement of aleuriospores

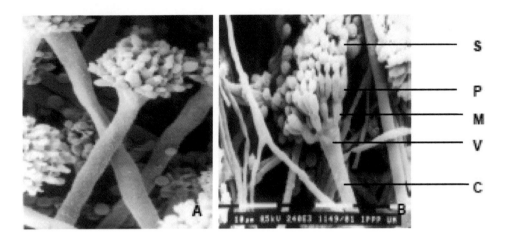

S= Aleuriospores , P= Phialides, M= Metulae, V= Vesicle, C= Conidiophore

Figure 13. Aleuriospores and associated structures of *Penicillium* species

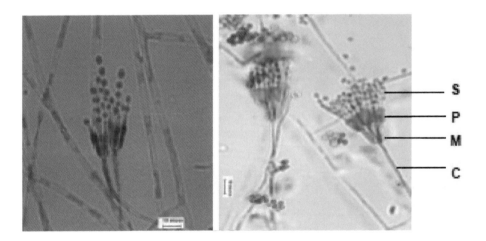

S= Aleuriospores , P= Phialides, M= Metulae, C= Conidiophore

The spores of dematiaceous fungi are formed at the enlarged tip of a stalk-like conidiophore or phialides. These spores bud to form spores at their distal end. The process continues until branching chains of conidia are formed with the youngest spores at the end.

The types of sporulations in dematiaceos fungi:

1. Phialophora-type sporulation: a flask-shaped phialide with the terminal end having a flared lip around the opening from which conidia are extruded (Fig. 14A).

2. Rhinocladiella-type sporulation: a conidiophore that develops terminally or along mycelium, the conidiophore develops into a swollen roughened appearance from which conidia develop along the length and terminus of the conidiophore (Fig. 14B).
3. Cladosporium-type sporulation: conidiophore with terminal or lateral ramifications producing branched conidial chains (Fig. 14C).

Figure 14. Types of sporulation for the identification of dematiaceous fungi

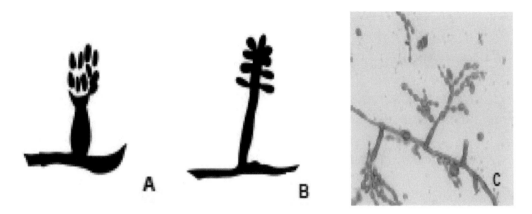

In Zygomycetes: sporangiospores (endospores) are developed inside a swollen, cellophane-like structure called a sporangium that is developed on a hypha, or a branch called a sporangiophore (Fig. 15).

Figure 15. Sporulation with large sporangium, sporangiophore and aseptate hyphae in Zygomycetes

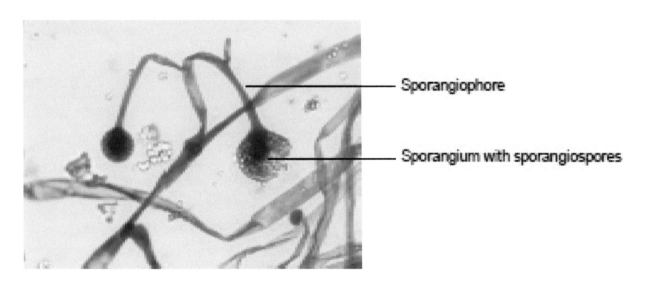

Section 2. Laboratory Diagnosis of Fungal Infections

Sample collection

- All samples for mycological investigation must be collected in a sterile container.
- The type of specimen depends on clinical presentation. It can be skin scraping, nail clipping, hair, sputum, tissue or caseous material, body fluids, or urine.
- For fungal blood culture, the blood is collected in commercially prepared blood culture bottles.

Direct microscopic examination

- Clinical samples are treated with 40% KOH that causes keratin cells to swell and reveal the fungal elements in the skin or nails (Fig. 16).

Stains commonly used in the Mycology laboratory

- Lactophenol Cotton Blue stain: Cotton Blue is an acid dye that stains the chitin in fungal cell walls.
- India ink: India ink contains carbon black particles that block out all the light except for the polysaccharide coating produced by fungi or bacteria. This is used in the mycology laboratory principally for identifying the capsule of *Cryptococcus neoformans* (Fig. 17A).
- Gomori's methenamine silver nitrate stain (GMS): This causes the cell wall to appear dark due to the deposit of silver stain (Fig. 17B).

Figure 16. Direct microscopic examination of clinical specimens with unique mycological presentations

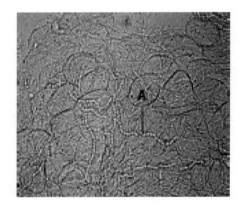

Dermatophytes: segmented, branching mycelial elements, may or may not break up into arthrospores (A)

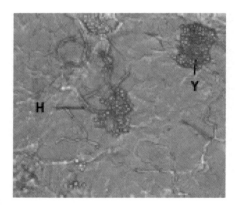

Malassezia furfur: cluster of round budding yeast cells (Y) and short fragments of septate hyphae (H)

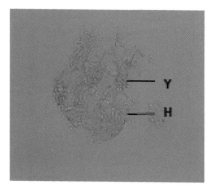

Malassezia furfur: cluster of round budding yeast cells (Y) and short fragments of septate hyphae (H)

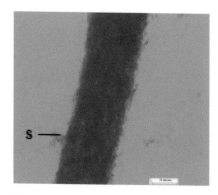

Ectothrix: hair invasion by dermatophytes *(M. canis, T. mentagrophytes).* Dermatophytes break out of the surface of the hair and break up to spores (S)

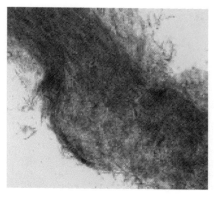

Endothrix type hair invasion: hair becomes fragile and breaks off, caused by dermatophytes (*T. violaceum, T. tonsurans*)

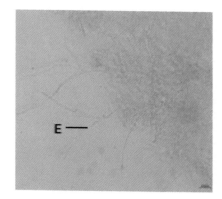

Direct microscopic examination of nail cutting after KOH treatment: detection of fungal elements (E)

Figure 17. Direct microscopic examination of specimens using India ink (A) and Gomori's methenamine silver nitrate stain (B)

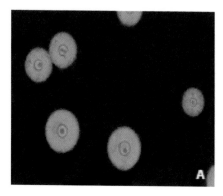

Cryptococcus neoformans: encapsulated yeast cells

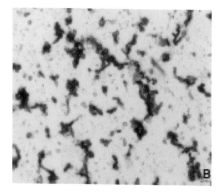

The fungal cell wall appeared dark due to the deposition of silver stain

Cultural procedures

Morphology is primarily used to establish the genus of the fungus; some fungal isolates can be identified to the species level.

Sabouraud Dextrose Agar (SDA) is the culture medium commonly used in the laboratory. The plate may have to be covered with olive oil if *Malassezia furfur* is suspected.

The wet-mount or tease-mount technique is widely used in the mycology laboratory for preparing fungal (mould) colonies for microscopic examination.

The slide-culture technique (Fig. 18) permits the microscopic observation of the undisturbed arrangement of spores and hyphae. This technique is important for the identification of filamentous fungi but not yeast-like fungi.

Figure 18. Slide-culture technique applied in the mycology laboratory

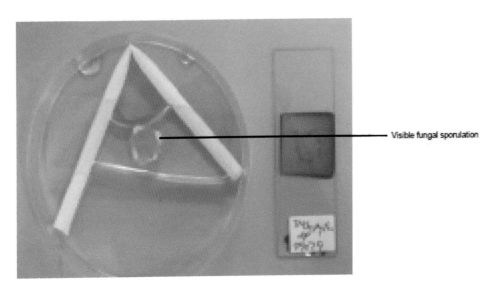

Visible fungal sporulation

A. Laboratory procedures for the identification of yeast-like fungi
The laboratory algorithm for identification of yeast-like fungi is different from that for moulds. For identification of yeast-like fungi, potato dextrose agar or Cornmeal-Tween 80 agar may be needed to stimulate the production of chlamydospores or blastospores.

- Describe the characteristics (colour, texture, and topography) of the colony (Fig. 19).
- Confirm the yeast-like cells by performing a gram stain (Fig. 3).
- Differentiate *Candida* species and *Cryptococcus* species by urease test.

   - A urease test negative is most likely *Candida* species; further identification of the *Candida* species is described in the respective section.
   - A urease test positive could be *Cryptococcus* or *Trichosporon* species. Refer to the respective sections for further identification.

Figure 19. Preliminary identification of yeasts by culture characteristics on SDA

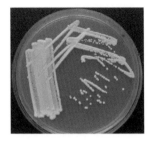 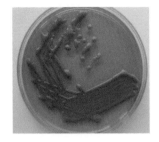 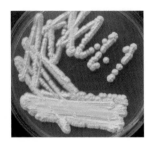 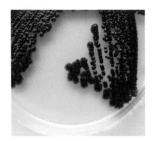

B. Laboratory procedures for the identification of moulds
Both a wet mount and slide-culture are required for the microscopic examination of a fungal culture.

- Describe the cultural characteristics (colour, texture, and topography) of the colony (Fig. 20).
- Prepare a Lactophenol Cotton Blue wet mount to study the microscopic morphologies of the moulds.
- Prepare a slide-culture for better demonstration of the microscopic features (Fig. 21).

Figure 20. Preliminary identification of mould culture on SDA

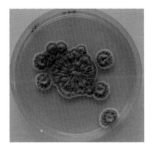 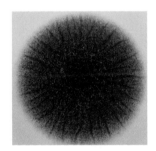 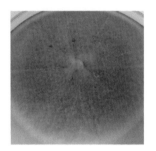 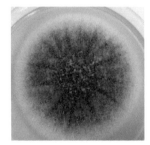

Figure 21. Cultural identification of moulds based on the characteristics of the asexual spores

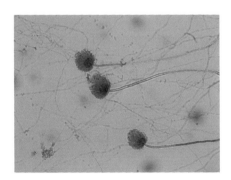 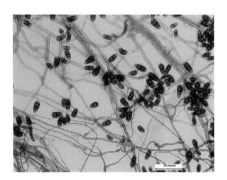

Aspergillus species: distinctive conidial heads with vesicles, phialides, and conidia. The conidiophores are long and have a smooth surface

Bipolaris species: septated hyphae, conidiophores unbranched, regularly geniculated. Conidia cylindrical with round ends, 3-distoseptate

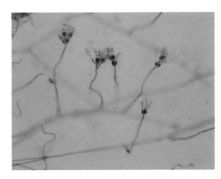

Penicillium species: branched conidiophores, phialides with chains of conidia

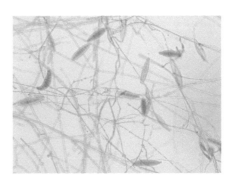

Microsporum species: spindle-shaped macroconidia

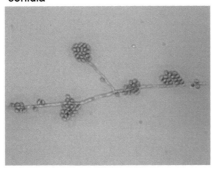

Sporothrix species: short conidiogenous cells arising from septated hyphae, conidia single-celled clustered at tip or side with denticles

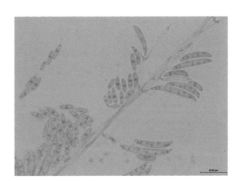

Fusarium species: branched conidiophores may form in clusters, macroconidia narrow sickle-shaped with transversed septa; beaked apical and pedicellated basal cells

Biochemical tests

Biochemical tests are used to differentiate the yeast-like fungi, especially the *Candida* and *Cryptococcus* species.

The carbohydrate assimilation test is based on the capability of the yeasts to assimilate the different types of carbon sources.

The carbohydrate assimilation test can be prepared in the laboratory using carbon-free base agar and filter paper discs impregnated with various carbohydrates (Table 4). The organism is cultured on the carbon free base agar with carbohydrate discs and incubated at 30°C for 24-48 hours (Fig. 22).

Table 4. Types of carbohydrate discs used for biotyping of *Candida* species and other yeast-like fungi

Candida sp. (Germ tube positive)	*Candida* sp. & other yeasts
Xylose	*Glucose*
α-methyl-D-glucoside	*Sucrose*
	Trehalose
	Maltose
	Galactose
	Cellobiose
	Arabinose

Figure 22 . Carbohydrate assimilation test prepared in the laboratory (A) and commercial API 20 C AUX system (B)

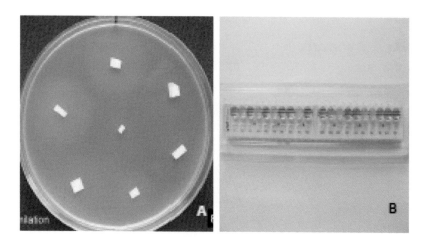

The carbohydrate assimilation test can be performed using the commercial API 20 C AUX system. The system consists of 20 cupules containing dehydrated substrates, which enable the performance of 19 assimilation tests. The cupules are inoculated with a semi-solid minimal medium, and the yeasts will only grow in cupules if they are capable of utilizing each substrate as the sole carbon source.

The reactions are read by comparing them to the controls, and identification is obtained by referring to the analytical profile index or using identification software.

Molecular identification of fungus

The molecular identification approach, particularly Polymerase Chain Reaction (PCR), is now widely used in the laboratory as an additional method to complement phenotypic or morphological approaches in accurate fungal species identification. The International Sub-commission on Fungal Barcoding has proposed the ribosomal Internal Transcribed Spacer (ITS) region as the prime fungal molecular marker for species identification. Many other markers have been designed and extensively used for specific purposes such as: subunit of RNA Polymerase genes RPB1 & RPB2, D1/D2 large subunit rDNA gene, and β-tubulin.

The workflows of ITS1-5.8s and RNA-ITS2 ribosomal RNA regions in fungal identification include harvesting the fungal culture on a medium, DNA extraction, PCR amplification, gel electrophoresis of amplified DNA (Fig. 23) followed by subsequent amplicon purification. Purified amplicons are subsequently prepped for cycle sequencing where sequencing primers, deoxynucleosidetriphosphates (dNTPs), and DNA polymerase are linearly amplified and subjected to dye terminator sequencing (Fig. 24).

Raw data from the process of dye terminator sequencing in the form of chromatograms are subjected to quality assessment and trimming to eliminate sequencing errors using suitable cutoff values. Cleaned amplicons from corresponding primer pairs are then assembled and subsequently subjected to phylogenetic analysis. This analysis involves data mining of suitable comparative species from publicly available database such as the NCBI to obtain a list of possible IDs based on the similarity of the unknown isolate to the reference sequences on the NCBI database. Data-mined datasets should be aligned using multiple sequence alignment tools such as Clustal W, Clustal X, or MUSCLE.

Phylogenetic tree (Fig. 25) construction using the appropriate substitution models and matrices is conducted using the finalized alignments to obtain the taxonomic position of the species.

Figure 23. The workflow of molecular identification of fungus

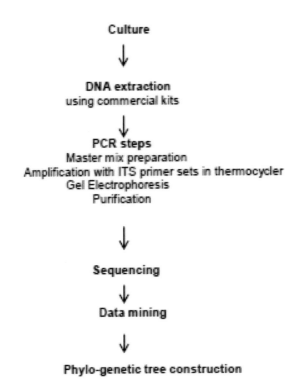

Figure 24. Gel electrophoresis of amplified fungal DNA

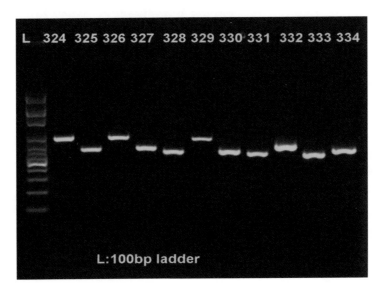

Fig 25. Phylogenetic tree of fungal DNA sequences with reference sequences from NCBI database

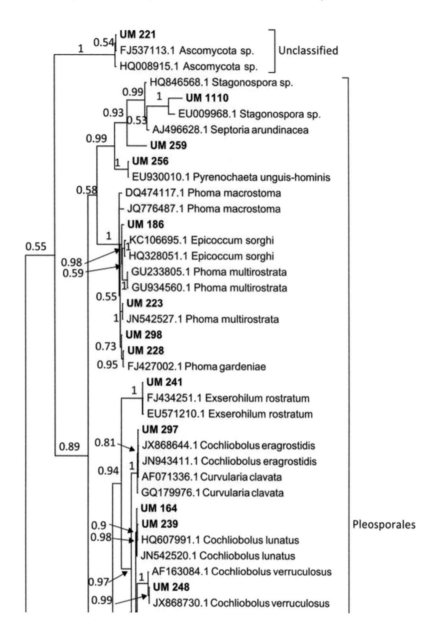

Histopathology examinations

Histopathology is an important diagnostic tool in mycology. It is cheap and provides a rapid presumptive identification of the infecting fungus. Some fungi cannot be cultivated in the laboratory, e.g. *Rhinosporidium seeberi* and *Pneumocystis jirovecii*. The diagnosis of the infections is derived from the histopatholgical examination of clinical specimens.

Figure 26. Histopathological examination of tissues with mycological pathognomonic diagnostic characteristics

A,B&C: *Cryptococcus neoformans*: yeast-like cells, variable in size and shape; few single budding cells. The yeast cells are separated by a clear space originally occupied by capsule (C). The spiny appearance of the capsular material is due to shrinkage and loss of mucicarmine-positive capsular materials.

D: *Histoplasma capsulatum*: the intracellular yeast cells within the histiocytes of bone marrow.

E: *Sporothrix schenckii*: asteroid body (A), large and small forms, typical elongated (cigar-shape) cells and the presence of hyphae bearing conidia. Budding yeast cells, usually multiple buddings, can be seen.

F,G&H: *Penicillium marneffei*: the yeast cells do not bud; equal cells with a transverse septum (H).

I: *Pneumocystis jirovecii (Pneumocystis carinii)*: presence of cup-shaped or hat-shaped forms, small round structure with thick wall.

J&K: *Aspergillus*: septate hyphae with streaming or parallel walls, repeated, dichotomous branching and vesicles.

L,M&N: *Candida* species: the presence of budding yeast-like cells, pseudomycelium, occasionally septate hyphae. *Candida glabrata* (N) produces only budding yeast-like cells.

O,P&Q: Zygomycosis: aseptated hyphae, broad, thin-walled, non-parallel and irregularly branched, and non-homogenous stained segments.

R: Phaeohyphomycosis: thick-walled oblong conidial chains, septated hyphae, possible fungus: *Phialophora* species, *Exophiala* species, *Cladosporium* species.

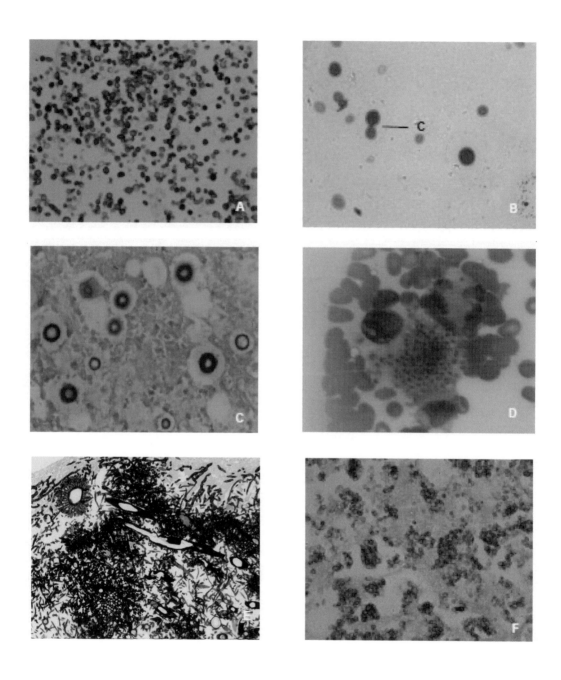

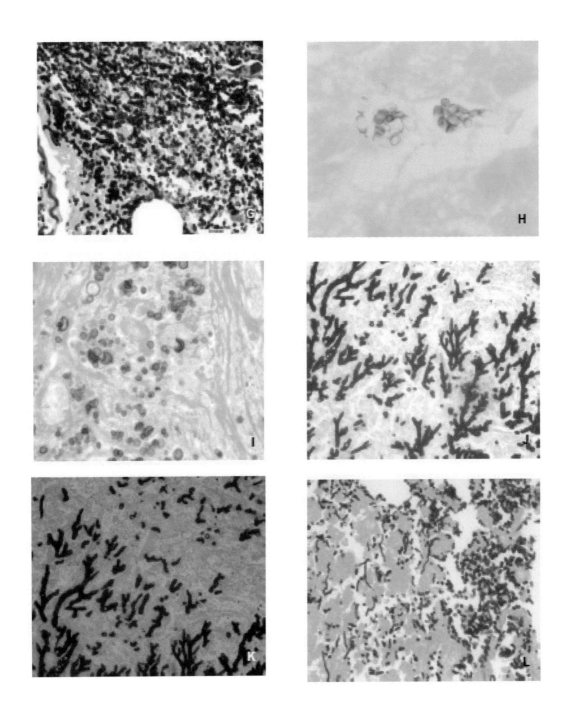

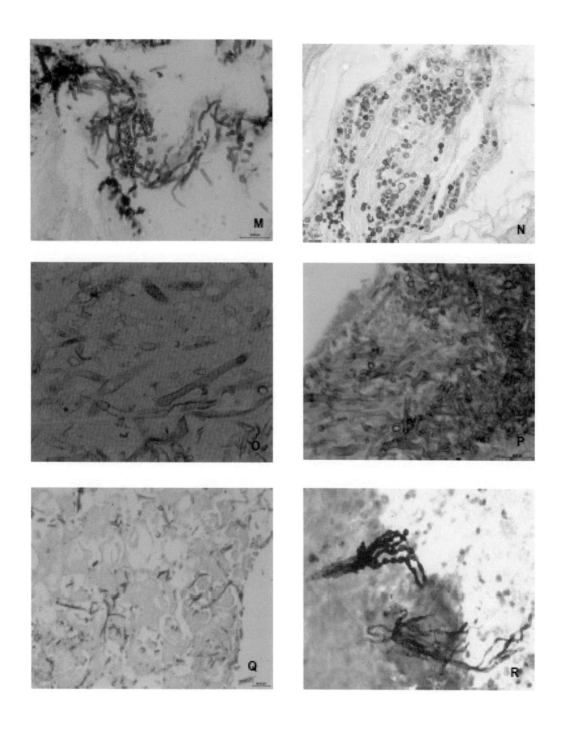

Section 3. Yeasts and Yeast-like Fungi

Yeasts are unicellular organisms reproduced by budding. Yeasts may produce pseudohyphae or true hyphae, but some do not produce hyphae at all.

The majority of the medically important yeast-like fungi such as *Candida* and *Trichosporon* produce true hyphae or pseudohyphae. *Saccharomyce*s are known as true yeasts as they do not produce either true hyphae or pseudohyphae.

All yeasts and yeast-like fungi grow on SDA (Fig. 27A). The identification of these fungi is based on the production of true hyphae or pseudohyphae or chlamydospore formation and their capability to utilize various sugars by assimilation.

The group consists of the following clinically important organisms:

> *Candida* species
> *Cryptococcus* species
> *Trichosporon* species
> *Rhodotorula* species
> *Malassezia* species
> *Geotrichum* species
> *Ustilago* species

Microscopic examination of yeasts and yeast-like fungi
> Gram stain:
>> *Candida* species: yeast-like, 4-8 ựm, budding, psedomycedium present or absent.
>> *Cryptococcus* species: yeast-like, budding, no pseudomycelium.
>> *Trichosporon* species: budding yeast cells, arthroconidia, meristematic cells often formed.
>> *Geotrichum* species: hyphae hyaline and branched, arthroconidia.

Candida species

- They are characterized by globose to elongated yeast-like cells or blastoconidia that reproduce by multilateral budding (Fig. 27B).
- All *Candida* species assimilate glucose as a carbon source.
- Most *Candida* species produce pseudohyphae, however this characteristic is absent in *Candida glabrata*.
- Clinical manifestations include oral thrush, systemic infections in immunocompromised patients (Fig. 27C).
- Yeast-like fungi on culture and in tissue appear as filamentous (pseudomycelium) and unicellular oval or spherical budding cells (Fig. 27D).

Figure 27. *Candida* species on SDA (A), stained by gram stain (B), oral thrush (C), and tissue with *Candida* infection (D)

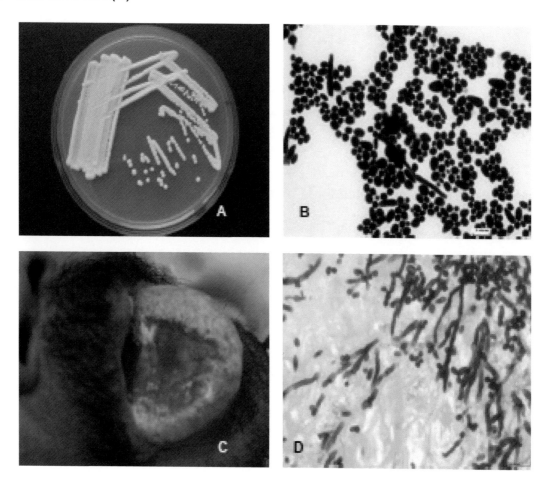

Habitat

- normal flora of man.
- found in the gut, uterus/vagina, and oral cavity.

Laboratory Identification

1. Germ-tube test: if positive → *Candida albicans, Candida dubliniensis*
   if negative → non-albicans *candida*

   Germ-tube production method

   1. Suspend the yeast cells in serum.
   2. Incubate the suspension at 35°C for 2.5 to 3 hours.
   3. Place a drop of the suspension on a clean microscope slide.
   4. Place a clean cover glass over the suspension, and then examine under low-power and high-power objective to confirm the presence or absence of germ-tubes (Fig. 29D).

2. Chlamydospore production on Cornmeal-Tween 80 agar.

   Chlamydospores are produced by *Candida* species and many filamentous fungi. They can be terminal or intercalary (Fig. 9).

3. Sugar assimilation patterns

   Bases on carbon free base medium impregnated with different types of sugars (Fig. 22A).

4. API 20C AUX system

   Commercial test system, procedures recommended by the manufacturer (Fig. 22B).

5. Chromogenic medium

   This medium can be used for a presumptive identification of *Candida albicans* (Fig. 28A), *Candida krusei*, and a few medically important *Candida* species. The medium is also useful for the detection of mixed *Candida* species infections (Fig. 28B).

Figure 28. Application of chromogenic medium for differentiating *Candida* species (A) and detection of mixed *Candida* species infections (B)

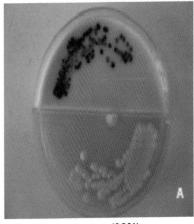

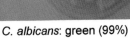

C. albicans: green (99%)

Important species isolated in the laboratory

Candida albicans	*Candida dubliniensis*
Candida krusei	*Candida parapsilosis*
Candida tropicalis	*Candida glabrata*
Candida rugosa	*Candida guilliermondii*
Candida lusitaniae	*Candida haemulonii*

Candida albicans

- Grows rapidly; colonies are white to cream, smooth, or glistening (Fig. 29A). Some variants may show dry and wrinkled colonies.
- Microscopic morphology shows round or short-oval budding cells (Fig. 29B). Growth at 45°C, produce terminal chlamydospores (Ch), pseudomycelium (Ps) present, blastoconidia (Bl) arranged in cluster on Cornmeal-Tween 80 agar (Fig. 29C).
- Produces germ-tubes, formed in serum incubated at 35°C for 2.5-3 hours (Fig. 29D).
- Assimilates xylose and α-methyl-D-glucoside.

Figure 29. *Candida albicans*: macroscopic characteristics (A), gram stained smear (B), chlamydospore production (C) and germ-tube production (D)

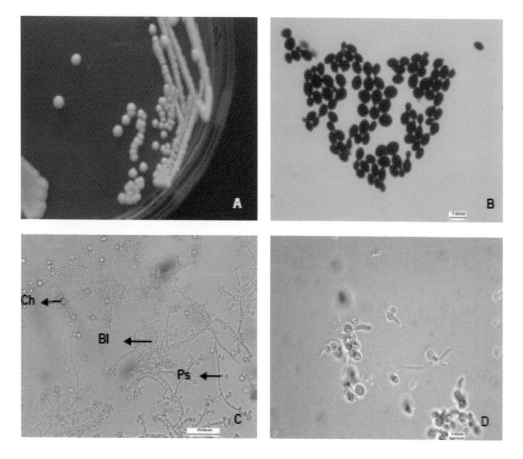

Carbohydrate assimilation characteristics of *Candida albicans*

Growth T °C			CHO Assimilation								
37	42	45	Glu	Suc	Tre	Mal	Gal	Cell	Arab	Xyl	α-D-glu
+	+	+	+	+	+	+	+	+	-	+	+

Glucose: Glu Sucrose: Suc Trehalose: Tre Maltose: Mal Galactose: Gal Cellobiose: Cell
Arabinose: Arab Xylose: Xyl α-methyl-D-glucoside : α-D-glu

Candida dubliniensis

- Grows rapidly, colonies are white to cream coloured, indistinguishable from *Candida albicans*, absence of growth at 45ºC.
- Microscopic morphology shows round or short-oval budding cells.
- On Cornmeal-Tween 80 agar, produces mostly terminal chlamydospores in chains of 1-3 or triplet terminal chlamydospores, pseudomycelium present, blastoconidia arranged in clusters (Fig. 30A).
- Produces germ-tubes (Fig. 30B).
- Does not assimilate xylose and α-methyl-D-glucoside.

Figure 30. *Candida dubliniensis:* chlamydospore production (A) and germ-tube production (B)

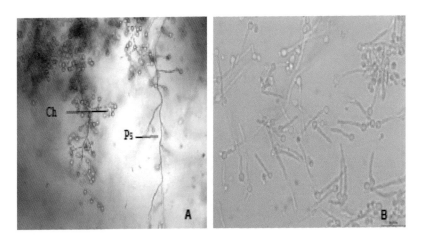

Carbohydrate assimilation characteristics of *Candida dubliniensis*

Growth T ºC			CHO Assimilation								
37	42	45	Glu	Suc	Tre	Mal	Gal	Cell	Arab	Xyl	α-D-glu
+	±	-	+	+	-	+	+	-	-	-	-

Candida krusei

- Colonies are flat, white or cream coloured, and smooth to dry.
- Microscopic morphology shows ellipsoidal to cylindrical budding yeast-like cells (Fig. 31A).
- Produces branched pseudomycelium, parallel with ovoid blastoconidia budding off from the verticilate branches on Cornmeal-Tween 80 agar (Fig. 31B).
- Assimilates only glucose.

Figure 31. *Candida krusei:* gram stained smear (A) and branched pseudomycelium (B)

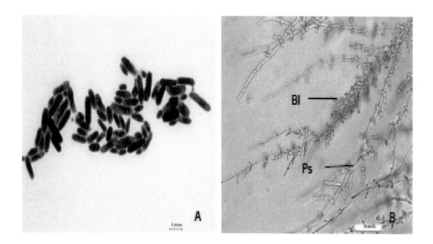

Carbohydrate assimilation characteristics of *Candida krusei*

Growth T °C			CHO Assimilation								
37	42	42	Glu	Suc	Tre	Mal	Gal	Cell	Arab	Xyl	α-D-glu
+	+	+	+	-	-	-	-	-	-	-	-

Candida parapsilosis

- Colonies are cream to yellow in colour, mostly smooth and glistening.
- Germ-tube test negative.
- Microscopic morphology shows round oval and long pseudomyedial cells (Fig. 32A).
- On Cornmeal-Tween 80 agar, abundant pseudomycelia arranged in Christmas tree-like pattern with blastoconidia scattered along the pseudomycelia. The branches are shorter at the apex of the pseudomycelium (Fig. 32B).
- Does not assimilate xylose, α-methyl-D-glucoside and cellobiose.

Figure 32. *Candida parapsilosis:* gram stained smear (A) and Christmas tree-like pseudomycelium (B)

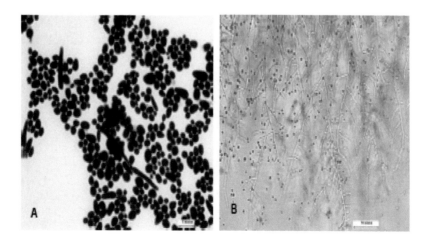

Carbohydrate assimilation characteristics of *Candida parapsilosis*

Growth T °C			CHO Assimilation								
37	42	45	Glu	Suc	Tre	Mal	Gal	Cell	Arab	Xyl	α-D-glu
+	+	+	+	+	+	+	+	-	-	-	-

Candida tropicalis

- Colonies are white to cream coloured, smooth and glistening (Fig. 33A).
- Microscopic morphology shows ellipsoidal budding cells with abundant pseudomycelium (Fig. 33B).
- Germ-tube test negative.
- On Cornmeal-Tween 80 agar, pseudomycelia poorly branched, clusters of ovoid blastoconidia grouped around the bases of pseudomycelium (Fig. 33C).
- Assimilates xylose and α-methyl-D-glucoside.

Figure 33. *Candida tropicalis:* colonies on SDA (A), gram stained smear (B) and branched pseudomycelium (C)

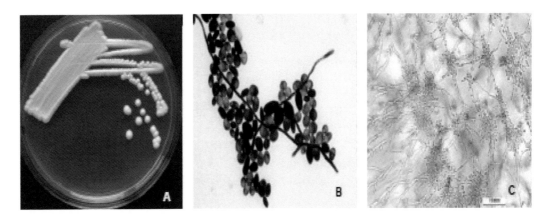

Carbohydrate assimilation characteristics of *Candida tropicalis*

Growth T °C			CHO Assimilation								
37	42	45	Glu	Suc	Tre	Mal	Gal	Cell	Arab	Xyl	α-D-glu
+	+	+	+	+	+	+	+	+	-	+	+

Candida glabrata

- Colonies are small, white, shiny and smooth.
- Ellipsoidal unipolar budding cells are typically arranged in dense groups (Fig. 34A).

- On Cornmeal-Tween 80 agar, no pseudomycelium, only small, oval, single blastoconidia (Fig. 34B).
- Assimilates trehalose.

Figure 34. *Candida glabrata:* gram stained smear (A) and single oval blastoconidia (B)

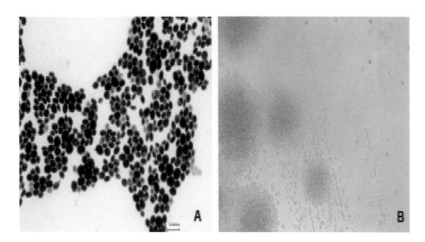

Carbohydrate assimilation characteristics of *Candida glabrata*

Growth T °C			CHO Assimilation								
37	42	45	Glu	Suc	Tre	Mal	Gal	Cell	Arab	Xyl	α-D-glu
+	+	+	+	-	+	-	-	-	-	-	-

Candida rugosa

- Colonies grow rapidly, are flat, white to creamy coloured, shiny and smooth or wrinkled.
- Produces no germ-tubes.
- Blastoconidia oval or elongate shaped, with long pseudomycelium (Fig. 35A).
- On Cornmeal-Tween 80 agar, small oval blastoconidia are clustered along the pseudohyphae (Fig. 35B).
- Assimilates galactose only.

Figure 35. Candida rugosa: gram stained smear (A) and oval blastoconidia on long pseudomycelium (B)

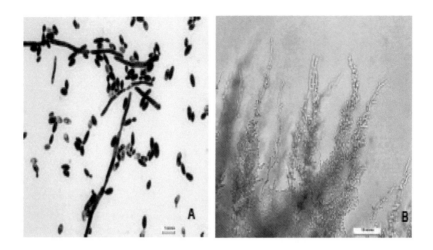

Carbohydrate assimilation characteristics of *Candida rugosa*

Growth	T °C					CHO Assimilation					
37	42	45	Glu	Suc	Tre	Mal	Gal	Cell	Arab	Xyl	α-D-glu
+	+	+	+	-	-	±	+	-	-	-	-

Cryptococcus species

- There are more than 30 different *Cryptococcus* species, but *Cryptococcus neoformans* causes nearly all cryptococcal infections in humans and animals.
- On SDA, the cultures are cream-coloured, mucoid or slimy in appearance (Fig. 36A).
- Microscopic morphology is characterized by globose to elongated yeast-like cells or blastoconidia that reproduce by multilateral budding (Fig. 36B).
- Pseudohyphae are absent.
- Most strains have capsules; the formation of a capsule is dependent on the culture medium. India ink stain demonstrates a distinct, wide, gelatinous capsule surrounding the yeast cells (Fig. 36C).
- Hydrolysed urea or urease is positive; fermentation of sugars is negative; assimilation of inositol is positive.
- On Cornmeal-Tween 80 agar, only the globose yeast cells are produced.
- In tissue, yeast-like cells are variable in size and shape, few single budding cells, no pseudomycelium (Fig. 36D).
- Important species: *Cryptococcus neoformans*, *Cryptococcus albidus*, *Cryptococcus laurentii*.

Figure 36. *Cryptococcus* species on SDA (A), gram stained smear (B), India ink (C) and in tissues (D)

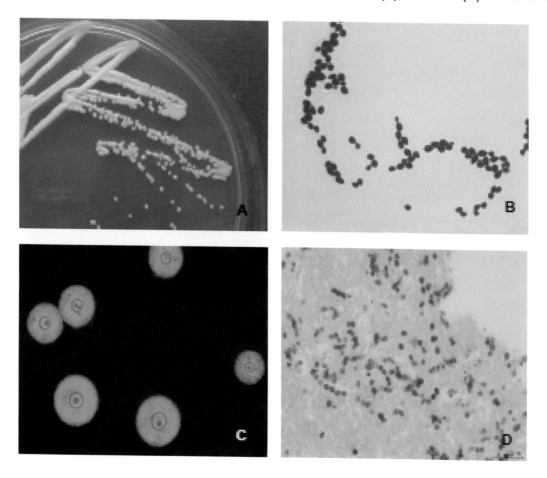

Cryptococcus neoformans

- It is traditionally divided into 2 varieties and 4 serotypes (A, B, C, D).
- *Cryptococcus neoformans var. neoformans* serotype A: *Cryptococcus neoformans var. grubii* and serotype D: *Cryptococcus neoformans* var. *neoformans*. Serotype A and serotype D are differentiated by molecular assay.
- *Cryptococcus neoformans var. gattii*: serotype B and C.
- The two varieties can be differentiated by Canavanine-glycine-bromthymol blue (CGB) agar (Fig. 37): *Cryptococcus neoformans var. gattii* isolates turn agar blue within 2-5 days. For *Cryptococcus neoformans var. neoformans* the colour of medium remains unchanged.

Figure. 37. Laboratory differentiation of two varieties of *Cryptococcus neoformans* by canavanine-glycin-bromthymol blue agar

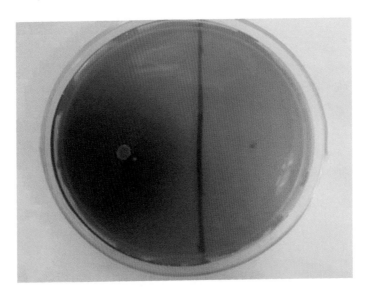

- Biochemical and physiological tests are important in identifying *Cryptococcus* species: growth at 37°C, lactose –, cellobiose –, melezitose +, nitrite – (Table 5).
- On Cornmeal-Tween 80 agar, yeast cells and multilateral budding yeast cells are seen; hyphae and pseudohyphae are absent (Fig. 38).

Figure 38. *Cryptococcus neoformans* var. *neoformans* on Cornmeal-Tween 80 agar

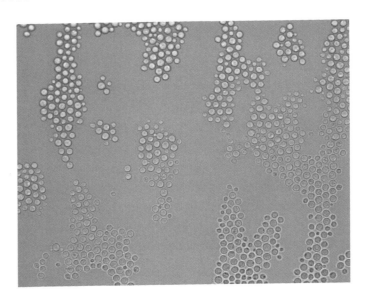

Cryptococcus albidus

- Colonies are glossy, slimy, and creamy white in colour (Fig. 39A).
- Yeast cells are spherical or ovoidal, single or multiple buddings (Fig. 39B).
- They produce no hyphae or pseudohyphae.
- Biochemical tests: sucrose +, maltose +, cellobiose +, nitrate + (Table 5).

Figure 39. *Cryptococcus albidus* on SDA (A) and gram stained smear (B)

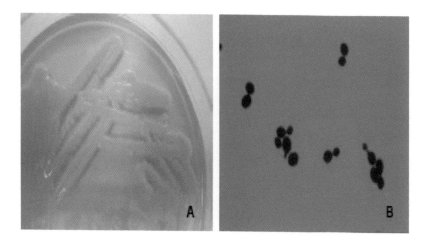

Cryptococcus laurentii

- Colonies are moist, mucoid or slimy, and creamy white in colour (Fig. 40A).
- Yeast cells are ellipsoidal, with multiple buddings (Fig. 40B).
- On Cornmeal-Tween 80 agar, no hyphae or pseudohyphae are produced.
- Test to differential from *Cryptococcus neoformans*: growth at 25°C but not at 37°C.

Figure 40. *Cryptococcus laurentii* on SDA (A) and gram stained smear (B)

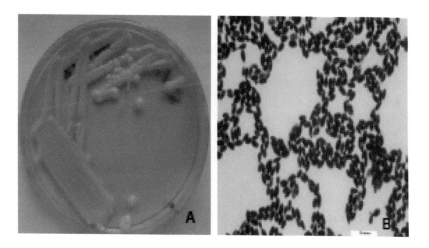

Table 5 Laboratory identification of *Cryptococcus* species by API method

Carbon	*Cryptococcus albidus*	*Cryptococcus neoformans*
D-Glucose	+	+
Glycerol	-	-
Calcium 2-Keto-Gluconate	+	+
L-Arabinose	+	-
D-Xylose	+	+
Adonitol	-	+
Xylitol	-	-
D-Galactose	-	+
Inositol	-	+
D-sorbitol	+	+
Methyl-D-Glucopyranoside	+	+
N-Acetyl-Glucosamine	-	+
D-Cellobiose	+	-
D-Lactose	-	-
D-Maltose	+	+
D-Saccharose	+	+
D-Trehalose	+	+
D-Melezitose	+	+
D-Raffinose	+	+

Positive: + Negative: -

Malassezia furfur

- Normal commensal of skin.
- Lipophilic yeast, growth must be stimulated by overlaying the Sabouraud Dextrose Agar (SDA) with olive oil (Fig. 41A).
- It is not possible to conduct usual sugar assimilation tests because of the lipid growth requirements.
- Budding yeast cells present, predominantly oval and some spherical cells (Fig. 41B).
- Causative agent of pityriasis versicolor (Fig. 41C).
- Direct microscopic examination of skin scraping shows yeast-like cells (Y) and pseudomycelium (H) (Fig. 41D).

Figure 41. *Malassezia furfur* on SDA (A), gram stained smear (B), pityriasis versicolor (C) and direct microscopic examination (D)

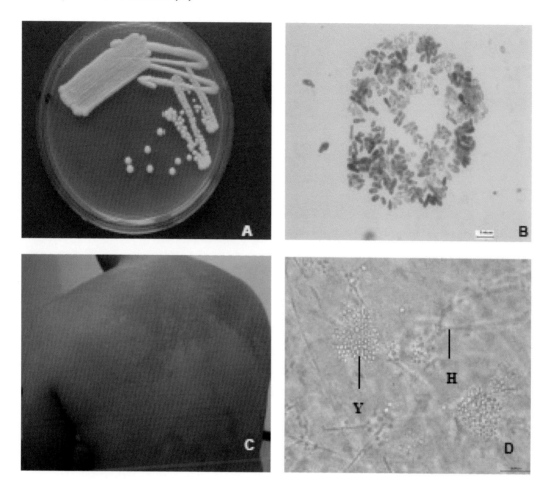

Trichosporon species

- Colonies are white, wrinkled, dry and dull in appearance with a mycelial fringe (Fig. 42A).
- Produce abundant pseudohyphae and some true hyphae segmenting into arthroconidia. Budding yeast-cells and blastoconidia present in chains or clusters (Fig. 42B).
- Identified by carbohydrate assimilation tests.
- Urease positive.

Figure 42. *Trichosporon* species on SDA (A) and gram stained smear (B)

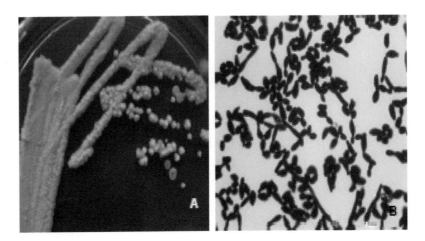

Geotrichum species

- Colonies grow rapidly, are flat, white to cream, with no reverse pigmentation (Fig. 43A).
- Hyphae septate, branched and break up into chains of arthroconidia (Fig. 43B).
- True blastoconidia and pseudohyphae are not found in this genus.
- The characteristic feature that distinguishes the genus *Geotrichum* from *Trichosporon* is the presence of blastoconidia, arthroconidia, and budding yeasts in the latter.
- Important species: *Geotrichum candidum.*

Figure 43. *Geotrichum* species on SDA (A) and gram stained smear (B)

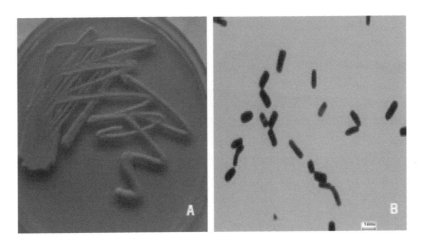

Rhodotorula species

- Colonies grow rapidly, are smooth, soft or mucoid, producing pink or reddish pigments (Fig. 44A).
- Do not ferment carbohydrates like *Candida* species; urease positive.
- Unicellular budding yeast cells, globose to elongated cylindrical shape, pseumycelium or hyphal elements absent (Fig. 44B).
- Important species: *Rhodotorula mucilaginosa.*

Figure 44. *Rhodotorula* species on SDA (A) and gram stained smear (B)

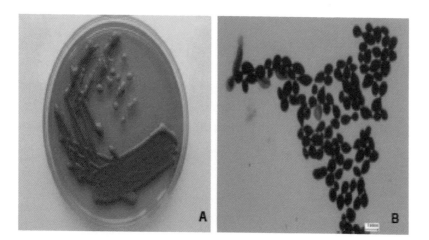

Ustilago species

- Colonies grow slowly and are moist and wrinkled. This organism is commonly found in soil and decaying vegetative material.
- In Lactophenol Cotton Blue stain, the blastoconidia are spindle-shaped, mixed with hyphae (Fig. 45A, B).
- Only one species: *Ustilago maydis*.

Figure 45. *Ustilago* species in Lactophenol Cotton Blue stain

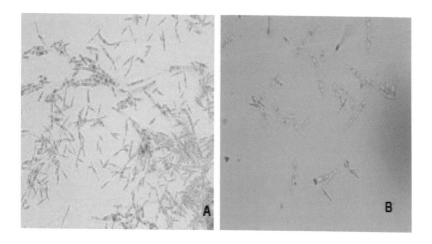

Section 4. Hyaline Hyphomycetes

- Hyaline hyphomycetes include filamentous fungi that do not produce dark pigments. The colonies may be white, green, or other colours.
- This group of fungi is identified by cultural characteristics (surface texture, topography, pigmentation), and microscopic features (conidial heads, type of conidia, arrangement/type of conidiogenous cells). The culture growth at different temperatures is also a criterion of identification.

Acremonium species

- Colonies are slow growing, cottony or compact and powdery, and initially white, becoming pale-pink (Fig. 46A).
- Septated hyphae, fine, long, simple, erect, and hyaline conidiogenous cells or phialides. Phialides taper towards apices.
- One-celled conidia, mostly aggregated in slimy head at the apex of each phialide (Fig. 46B).

Figure 46. The cultural and microscopic characteristics of *Acremonium* species

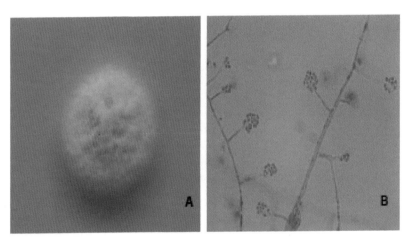

Aspergillus species

- Hyaline septated hyphae.
- Colonies are rapid growing, floccose, velvety to granular, woolly to cottony, and the colour may be white, yellow, yellow-brown, pink, brown to black, or shades of green.
- The genus is characterized by the conidiophore terminating in a swollen vesicle. The vesicle can be clavate, round, flask-shaped, covered with either a single layer of phialides/conidiogenous cells (uniseriate) or a layer of subtending cells (metulae) with whorls of phialides/conidiogenous cells on the top (biseriate) producing conidia.
- The arrangement of phialides or metulae on vesicles is an important identification feature.
- Conidia hyaline or pigmented, one-celled, smooth- or rough-walled, forming long divergent chains (radiate) or aggregated in compact columns (columnar).
- Conidial head is formed by the vesicle, metulae (if present), phialides, and conidia.
- Hülle cells or sclerotia may be found.

Aspergillus flavus

- Colonies grow rapidly; floccose, granular with radial grooves, initially white becoming yellow-green centrally with whitish edge with age (Fig. 47A).
- Conidial heads are typically radiate, biseriate, or uniseriate.
- Phialides or metulae cover the entire vesicles (Fig. 47B, C).
- Conidiophores are hyaline and coarsely roughened near the vesicles.
- Some strains produce brownish sclerotia.

Figure 47. The cultural and microscopic characteristics of *Aspergillus flavus*

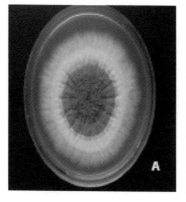 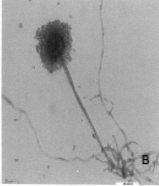 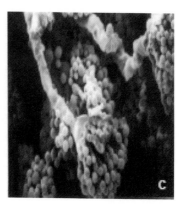

Aspergillus fumigatus

- Colonies grow rapidly; initially white, becoming blue-green in colour with characteristic terminally branched radial folds at the periphery of the colony (Fig. 48A).
- Conidiophores are short and broad, and the vesicles are conical-shaped with a single row of phialides on the upper two thirds of the vesicles (Fig. 48B, C).
- Conidial heads are typically columnar.
- Thermotolerant and grows at 55°C.

Figure 48. The cultural and microscopic characteristics of *Aspergillus fumigatus*

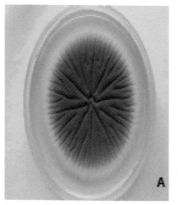 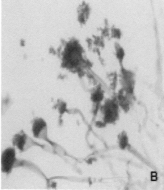 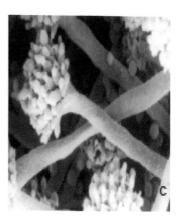

Aspergillus niger

- Colonies grow rapidly and are floccose and initially white. The surface becomes black due to a dense layer of black conidial heads. The compact basal and peripheral hyphae remain white (Fig. 49A).
- Conidiophores are small and smooth-walled with globose vesicles.
- Conidial heads are biseriate, radiate with conidia forming loose columns (Fig. 49B, C).
- This is the third most common species associated with invasive pulmonary aspergillosis, also a common laboratory contaminant.

Figure 49. The cultural and microscopic characteristics of *Aspergillus niger*

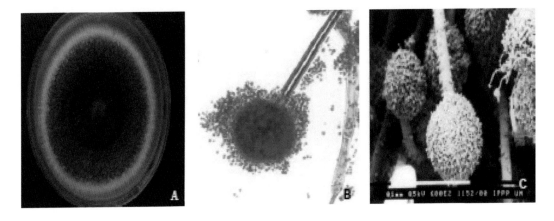

Aspergillus terreus

- Colonies grow rapidly and are floccose, sand-brown centrally with compact white mycelium peripherally, and branched radiate folds (Fig. 50A).
- Conidiophores hyaline, thin- and smooth-walled with ellipsoidal vesicles.
- Conidial heads are biseriate, the metulae located on the upper half of the vesicles (Fig. 50B).
- Conidia radiate, forming long compact columns.
- Used to produce organic acids; a known human opportunistic pathogen.

Figure 50. The cultural and microscopic characteristics of *Aspergillus terreus*

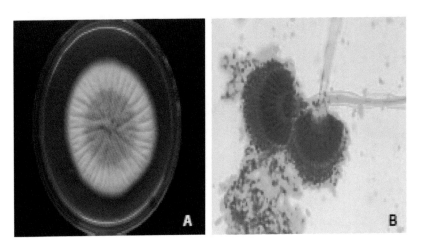

Aspergillus nomius

- Colonies grow rapidly and are floccose, white, with the center raised with rims of compact yellow and light-brown conidial heads (Fig. 51A).
- Conidiophores hyaline, rough-walled, and long.
- Vesicles small, ellipsoidal, biseriate; the conidiogenous cells cover the upper two thirds (Fig. 51B, C).
- Conidia heads are small and radiate, forming long, loose columns.

Figure 51. The cultural and microscopic characteristics of *Aspergillus nomius*

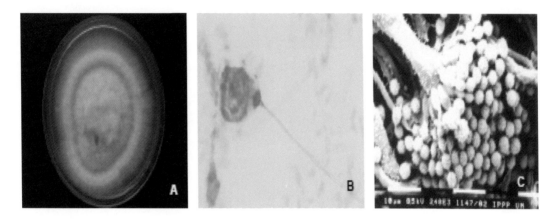

Aspergillus ustus

- Colonies grow rapidly and are velvety, with a raised center with radial groves, dull brown in colour (Fig. 52A).
- Conidiophores hyaline, long, and smooth-walled.
- Vesicles are globose to subspherical; conidiogenous cells are biseriate with metulae covering the upper half of the vesicles (Fig. 52B, C, D).
- Conidial heads are small and radiate, forming short, loose columns.

Figure 52. The cultural and microscopic characteristics of *Aspergillus ustus*

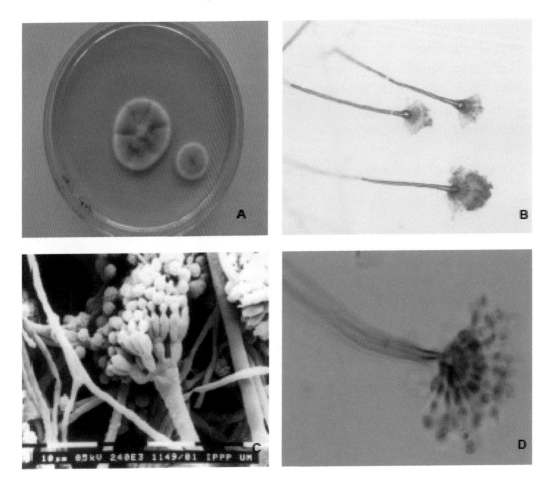

Aspergillus oryzae

- Colonies grow rapidly, are snow white in young culture, and become greenish-yellow with age (Fig. 53A).
- Conidiophores are hyaline, long, and rough-walled.
- Vesicles are subspherical; conidiogenous cells may be uniseriate or biseriate.
- Metulae or phialides cover the entire or upper three fourths of the vesicles (Fig. 53B, C, D).
- Conidial heads are small and radiate, forming loose columns.
- Used by the Chinese and Japanese to make rice vinegars and sake.

Figure 53. The cultural and microscopic characteristics of *Aspergillus oryzae*

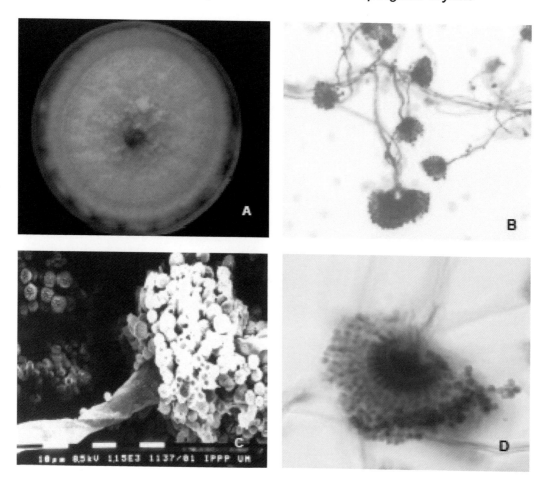

Aspergillus aculeatus

- Colonies grow rapidly and are felty, black centrally with shades of white and compact hyphae on the periphery (Fig. 54A).
- Reverse side on culture plate is brownish with radiating groves (Fig. 54B).
- Conidiophores are short, broad, smooth-walled, and slightly pigmented at the apex near the vesicles (Fig. 54C).
- Vesicles are subspherical; conidiogenous cells are uniseriate and cover the entire vesicles (Fig. 54C, D) .
- Conidial heads are radiate, forming well-defined columns.

Figure 54. The cultural and microscopic characteristics of *Aspergillus aculeatus*

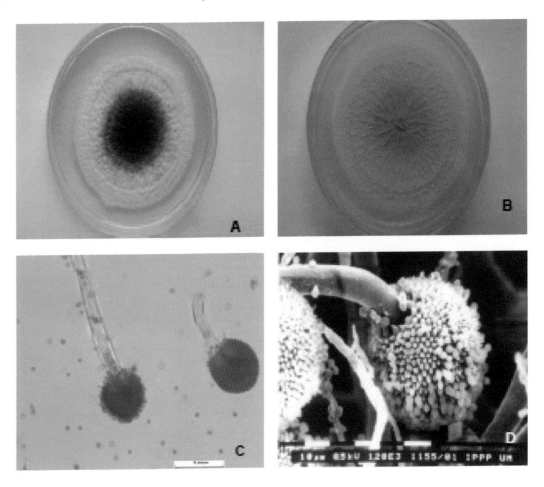

Aspergillus sydowii

- Colonies grow rapidly and spread with a central fold of compact aerial mycelium, blue-green in colour (Fig. 55A).
- Conidiophores are hyaline, long, and smooth-walled.
- Vesicles are subspherical; conidiogenous cells are biseriate, and cover the upper half of vesicles.
- Conidial heads are small and radiate, forming loose columns (Fig. 55B, C).
- Spherical Hülle cells may be present.

Figure 55. The cultural and microscopic characteristics of *Aspergillus sydowii*

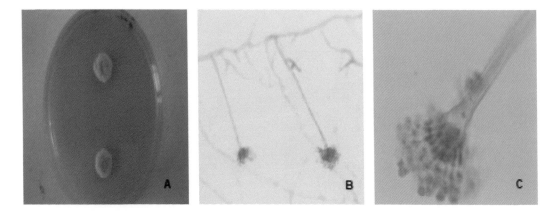

Paecilomyces species

- Colonies are fast growing, flat, woolly, and powdery or velvety in texture.
- Initially white, they become greyish-brown or tan depending on the species, but never green as in *Penicillium* (Fig. 56A).
- Phialides are swollen at their bases, gradually tapering into a long, slender neck, occurring solitarily or in pairs or as verticils or in penicillate heads. Long chains of single-celled conidia are produced from the phialides (Fig. 56B).
- The genus *Paecilomyces* may be distinguished from another closely related genus *Penicillium* by its long slender phialides and colonies that are never classically green.

Figure 56. The cultural and microscopic characteristics of *Paecilomyces* species

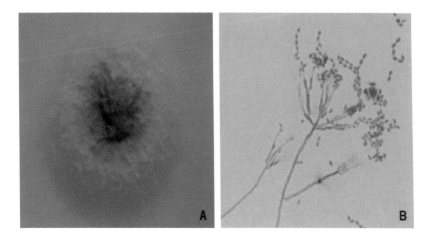

Paecilomyces variotii

- Colonies grow rapidly and are floccose to powdery, yellow-brown or sandy coloured centrally with white expanding mycelia (Fig. 57A).
- Conidiophores produce branches that are arranged verticillately or in whorls; each branch bears a phialide which is cylindrical in shape with a long tapering neck (Fig. 57B).
- Conidia ellipsoidal to fusiform, smooth-walled, arranged in long divergent chains.
- Chlamydospores are present.

Figure 57. The cultural and microscopic characteristics of *Paecilomyces variotii*

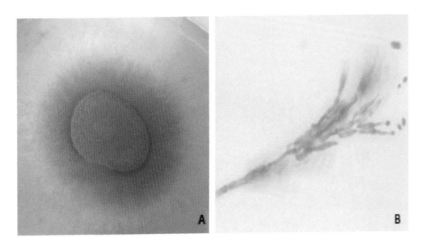

Chrysosporium species

- Colonies grow with moderate rapidity, and are flat, granular or woolly, and usually whitish (Fig. 58A).
- Hyphae septate, hyaline, smooth-walled, and branched (Fig. 58B).
- Conidia one-celled, hyaline, produced directly on the side branch or on a short protrusion of the hyphae. The conidia may be intercalary (Fig. 58C).
- Chlamydospores may be present (Fig. 58D).
- Important species isolated from clinical specimens: *Chrysosporium tropicum, Chrysosporium keratinophilum.*

Figure 58. The cultural and microscopic characteristics of *Chrysosporium* species

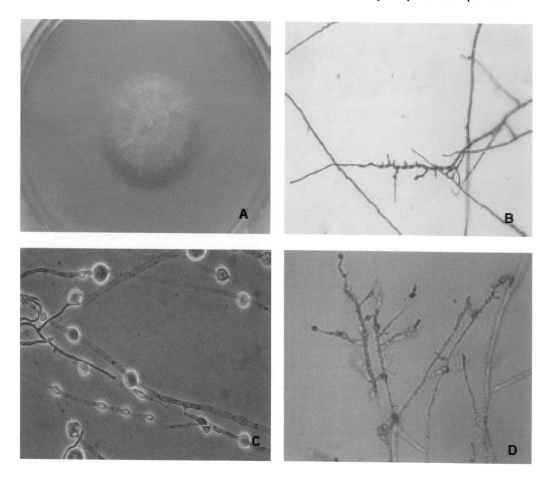

Scopulariopsis species

- Colonies grow rapidly and are initially white, light tan or brown; some species are black but never green. The texture may be velvety, powdery, or granular (Fig. 59A).
- Conidiophores are erect and short; annellated conidiogenous cells cluster forming a penicillus (Fig. 59B).
- Conidia round to ovoidal, rough-walled, and form basipetal chains.

Figure 59. The cultural and microscopic characteristics of *Scopulariopsis* species

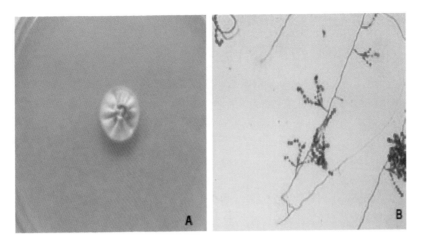

Scedosporium species

- Colonies grow rapidly and are initially white and cottony. They become flat with short aerial mycelium (Fig. 60A).
- Conidiophores are thin, short, single, or branched.
- Annellated conidiogenous cells are flask-shaped with swollen bases and tapering necks, arising directly from hyphae or formed at the tips of conidiophores.
- Conidia are unicellular, oval, and form clusters at the apices of the annellated conidiogenous cells (Fig. 60B).
- Two species: *Scedosporium apiospermum, Scedosporium prolificans.*

Figure 60. The cultural and microscopic characteristics of *Scedosporium* species

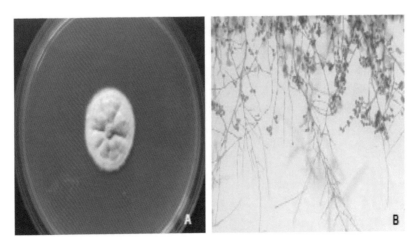

Trichoderma species

- Colonies grow rapidly and are cottony, initially white, and become granular with blue-green patches forming concentric rings (Fig. 61A).
- Hyaline septated hyphae with short conidiophores and phialides producing conidia.
- Phialides are flask-shaped with broad bases and narrow apices; they may be single or in clusters.

- Conidia one-celled, green in colour, spherical or ellipsoidal, may be smooth- or rough-walled, always grouped in the sticky heads at the narrow tips of phialides (Fig. 61B).

Figure 61. The cultural and microscopic characteristics of *Trichoderma* species

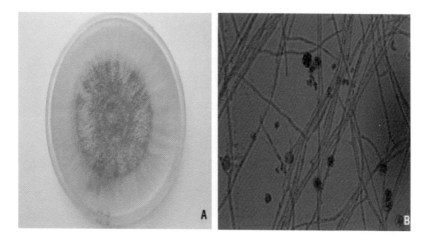

Sepedonium species

- Similar microscopic characteristics to *Histoplasma capsulatum* (Fig. 82), except for the lack of thermal dimorphism.
- On SDA plate incubated at 30°C, the colony is compact and initially white. At maturity the center becomes raised with light pink coloration (Fig. 62A).
- Large, rounded, single-celled, tuberculate macroconidia and small microconidia (Fig. 62B).

Figure 62. The cultural and microscopic characteristics of *Sepedonium* species

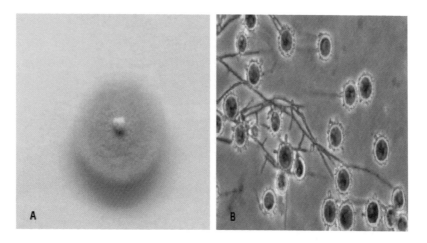

Penicillium species

- Colonies grow rapidly and are velvety, consisting of low compacted aerial mycelium. They are initially white and later become green, greenish-grey, or olive grey.
- Chains of single-celled conidia are produced by flask-shaped phialides.
- Phialides and metulae form a brush-like appearance commonly known as a penicillus.

- A branch refers to all cells (i.e. conidia, phialide) between the metulae and the stipes of conidiophores.
- Identification to the species level is based on the colonial morphology and microscopic patterns of branching (Fig. 63). The branches may be:
  - simple or monoverticillate (A)
  - one-stage branched or biverticillate-symmetrical (B)
  - two-stage branched or biverticillate-asymmetrical (C)
  - three- or more-stage branched (D)

- Sclerotia may be produced by some species.

Figure 63. Patterns of penicillus use in the identification of *Penicillium* species

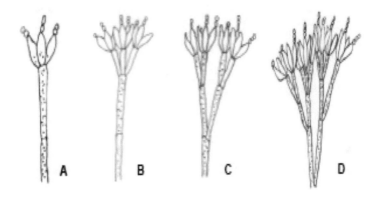

Penicillium marneffei

- Exhibits thermal dimorphism (Fig. 83); produces distinctive diffusible red-pigment around the colonies (Fig. 64A).
- Colonies grow rapidly; velvety in texture, initially white becoming granular and greenish yellow.
- Septated hyline hyphae; penicilli composed of branching biverticillate-symmetrical metulae and phialides which produce spherical conidia in chains (Fig. 64B).

Figure 64. The cultural and microscopic characteristics of *Penicillium marneffei*

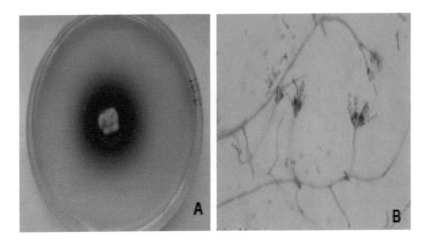

Penicillium corylophilum

- Colonies grow rapidly and are compact and granular with concentric rings of light-purple and green colour centrally. The mycelia are white peripherally (Fig. 65A).
- Conidiophores smooth-walled, long, biverticillate-symmetrical penicilli (Fig. 65B).

Figure 65. The cultural and microscopic characteristics of *Penicillium corylophilum*

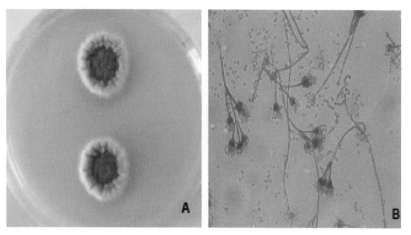

Penicillium citrinum

- Colonies grow rapidly, are velvety in texture, and are greyish-turquoise with prominent radial folds with a peripheral rim of white mycelium (Fig. 66A).
- White fluffy pigments are noted on the surface.
- Conidiophores short, smooth-walled, penicilli biverticillate-symmetrical, phialides flask-shaped with chains of spherical conidia (Fig. 66B).

Figure 66. The cultural and microscopic characteristics of *Penicillium citrinum*

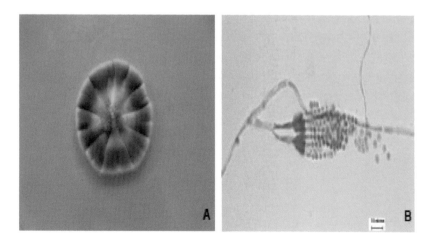

Penicillium fellutanum

- Colonies grow rapidly and are compact with short aerial mycelium, granular with greenish-grey center, and white short aerial mycelium peripherally (Fig. 67A).

- Conidiophores long, smooth walled and unbranched.
- Simple or monoverticillate penicillus (Fig. 67B, C).

Figure 67. The cultural and microscopic characteristics of *Penicillium fellutanum*

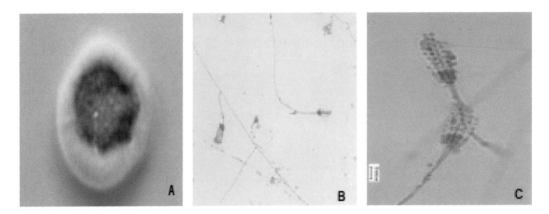

Fusarium species

- Colonies are usually fast growing, pale, grey, olive grey, or may be red coloured depending on the species.
- Produce both macro- and microconidia from slender phialides.
- Macroconidia are hyaline, two- to several-celled, fusiform- to sickle-shaped, mostly with an elongated apical cell and pedicellated basal cell.
- Microconidia are one- to two-celled, hyaline, pyriform, fusiform to ovoid, straight or curved.
- Chlamydoconidia may be present or absent.

Fusarium oxysporum

- Colonies grow rapidly and are initially white and purple or lavender at maturity (Fig. 68A).
- Hyphae are septated and hyaline. Conidiophores are short and unbranched.
- Macroconidia are slightly sickle-shaped thin-walled, 3-5 septate, apical cell attenuated and a foot-shaped basal cell (Fig. 68B, C).
- Microconidia abundant, single septum or non-septated, slightly curved or cylindrical shaped.
- Chlamydoconidia present singly or in pairs.

Figure 68. The cultural and microscopic characteristics of *Fusarium oxysporum*

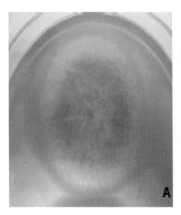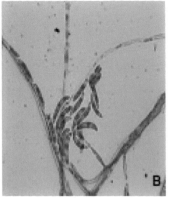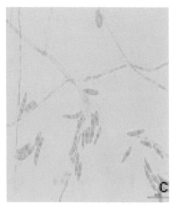

Fusarium solani

- Colonies grow rapidly and are initially white and floccose but become bluish-brown centrally with the formation of sporodochia, though the peripheral of the colonies remains creamy white (Fig. 69A).
- Conidiophores short and branched, bearing macroconidia. The macroconidia fusiform, slightly curved, thick walled, 3-5 septate with a short blunt apical cells (Fig. 69B).
- Microconidia abundant, oval to cylindrical, one to two cells, formed from a long monophialides (Fig. 69C, D).
- Chlamydospores hyline, globose, borne singly or in pairs, are abundant.

Figure 69. The cultural and microscopic characteristics of *Fusarium solani*

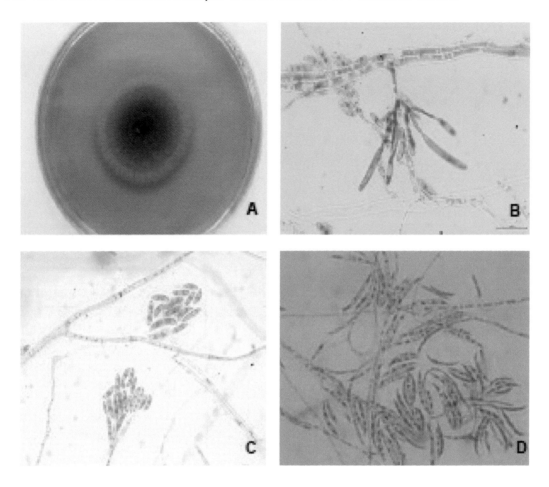

Fusarium nectroides

- Colonies grow rapidly and are initially white, becoming greyish-brown upon maturing, furrowed or vacuolated surface due to formation of sporodochia (Fig. 70A).
- Hyphae septated, macroconidia predominantly two-celled.
- Chlamydospores abundant, smooth-walled, single, or in pairs (Fig. 70B).

Figure 70. The cultural and microscopic characteristics of *Fusarium nectroides*

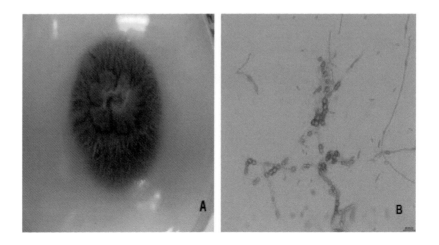

Section 5. Dermatophytes

- Consist of three genera which can be differentiated by the microscopic morphology of the micro and/or macroconidia.
- Known as keratinophilic fungi because they are able to grow on keratin such as hair, nail and skin. In humans, the disease caused by these fungi is generally known as ringworm or tinea (Fig. 71A, B, C, D).
- This group of fungi has never been reported as opportunistic pathogens.
- Can be antrophilic (human host), zoophilic (animal host) and geophilic (soils).

Figure 71. Common human infections caused by dermatophytes

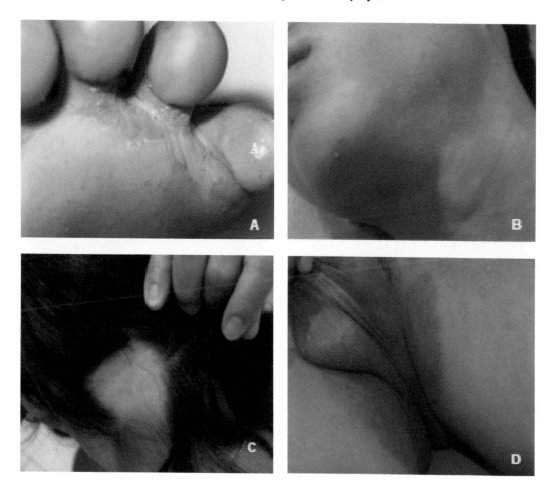

Epidermophyton species

- Colonies grow moderately rapidly, are green-brown to mustard-yellow in colour, initially flat becoming velvety with radial grooves (Fig. 72A).
- On the reverse side of culture plate, culture shows yellowish-tan.
- Macroconidia numerous; smooth thin-walled, club-shaped with blunt tip, no microconidia (Fig. 72B, C).
- Chlamydospore-like cells are abundant (Fig. 72D).

Figure 72. The cultural and microscopic characteristics of *Epidermophyton* species

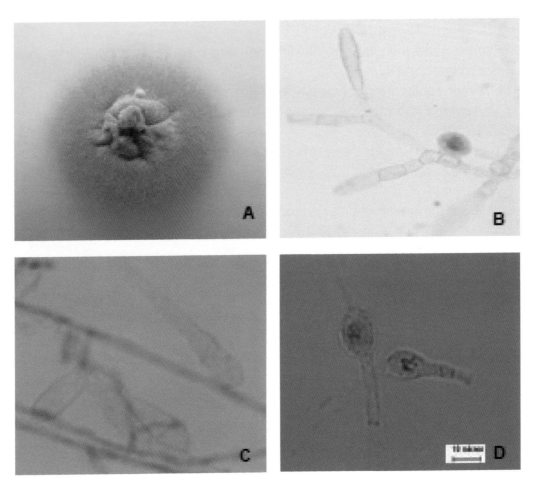

Microsporum species

- Colonies grow rapidly, are powdery or woolly with white to salmon tinges in colour. Reverse reddish or yellowish.
- Macroconidia present mostly solitarily alongside the septated hyphae. Macroconidia with rough walls or echinulate, spindle-shaped. Microconidia absent or rare, single, usually one-celled, ovoid, smooth-walled.
- *Microsporum* is the asexual state of the fungus; the telemorph phase is genus *Arthroderma*.

Microsporum canis

- Colonies grow rapidly and are spreading, woolly, initially white, brownish-yellow with concentric rings formation by aging (Fig. 73A).
- Reverse ochraceous-yellow.
- Macroconidia spindle-shaped, rough- and thick-walled with an asymmetrical apical knob, six to fifteen-celled with thin septal walls (Fig. 73B, C).
- Microconidia rare, unicellular and pyriform in shape sessile alongside the hyphae.

Figure 73. The cultural and microscopic characteristics of *Microsporum canis*

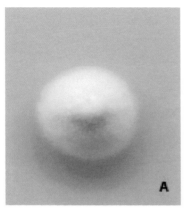 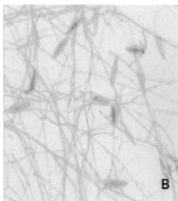 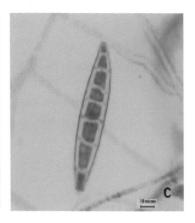

Microsporum gypseum

- Colonies grow rapidly, are flat or cottony with umbonated or central raised tufts, initially white becoming granular and cinnamon-tan (Fig. 74A).
- Macroconidia spindle-shaped, in cluster, thin or echinulate wall, 3-6 celled with round terminal cells, the basal cells truncated (Fig. 74B).
- Microconidia fusiform, sessile with smooth thin wall.

Figure 74. The cultural and microscopic characteristics of *Microsporum gypseum*

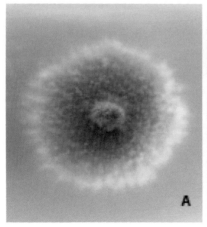 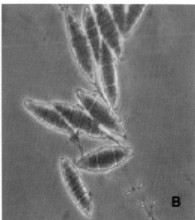

Trichophyton species

- Microconidia are predominantly one-celled, pyriform in shape, solitary, or in clusters.
- Macroconidia are smooth-walled, hyaline, multi-celled, and cigar- or pencil-shaped.
- Thallic macroconidia and microconidia, if present, are always arranged alongside undifferentiated hyphae.
- Important species: *Trichophyton mentagrophytes, Trichophyton rubrum, Trichophyton schoenleinii, Trichophyton verrucosum, Trichophyton violaceum.*

Trichophyton mentagrophytes

- Colonies grow moderately and are powdery with raised central tufts and radial folds, white to creamy (Fig. 75A).
- Macroconidia sparse, 3-8 celled, smooth walled and cigar-shaped (Fig. 75B).
- Microconidia are abundant, spherical, sessile, single, or arranged in grape-like clusters along the septated hyphae.
- Spiral hyphae and chlamydospores are present (Fig. 75C).

Figure 75. The cultural and microscopic characteristics of *Trichophyton mentagrophytes*

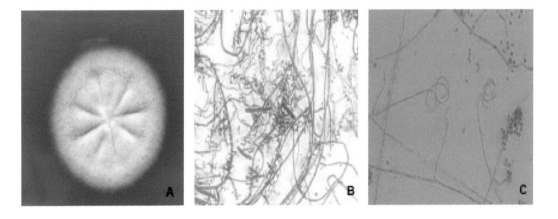

Trichophyton rubrum

- Colonies grow moderately and are cottony with raised central tufts, initially white becoming rose coloured (Fig. 76A).
- Macroconidia are sparse, cigar-shaped, multi-celled; wall is thin and smooth.
- Microconidia are abundant, fusiform, single, sessile, on the lateral side of hyphae, with some in clusters (Fig. 76B).

Figure 76. The cultural and microscopic characteristics of *Trichophyton rubrum*

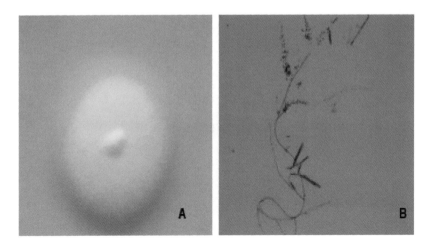

Section 6. Zygomycetes

- Colonies grow rapidly and are cottony and white to light grey in colour.
- Hyphae hyaline, broad and non-septated.
- They reproduce sexually by the fusion of undifferentiated isogametangia forming a thick-walled sexual structure called a zygospore.
- Asexual reproductions include long simple or branched sporangiophores bearing a sporangium containing sporangiospores. Some strains produce chlamydospores.
- Dome-like columella is present at the apex of sporangiophore in some species.
- Stolons bearing rhizoids may be present.
- The identification of the genus is based on the morphology and characteristics of asexual spores and the presence or absence of rhizoids.
- Two medically important orders:

  1. Mucorales: *Mucor, Rhizopus, Absidia, Rhizomucor, Cunninghamella, Syncephalastrum.*
  2. Entomophthorales: *Basidiobolus, Conidiobolus.*

- Species frequently isolated in the laboratory include: *Mucor, Rhizopus, Basidiobolus, Cunninghamella, Syncephalastrum.*

Mucor species

- Colonies grow rapidly and are cottony, initially white becoming dark grey (Fig. 77A).
- Hyphae are hyaline, broad and non-septated.
- Sporangiophores are long, erect, simple, or branched, bearing globose to spherical sporangium at the terminal; columellae are well developed but with no apophyses (Fig. 77B).
- Sporangiospores are hyaline, smooth-walled, and globose to ellipsoidal in shape.
- Stolons and rhizoids are absent.

Figure 77. The cultural and microscopic characteristics of *Mucor* species

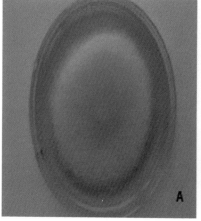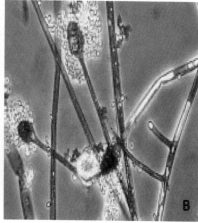

Rhizopus species

- Colonies are fast growing, initially white and cottony becoming brownish grey to blackish grey due to abundant sporangium (Fig. 78A).
- Hyphae are broad, hyaline, non-septated with stolons producing groups of sporangiophores and rhizoids.
- Sporangiophores arise from the opposite of rhizoids and stolons at the nodal region.
- Sporangiophores are smooth walled, simple, unbranched, and long, bearing globose sporangium; columella and apophysis are present at the apices of sporangiophores.
- Sporangiospores are subglobose to ellipsoidal; after releasing the spores, the sporangium collapses leaving an umbrella-like structure (Fig. 78B).

Figure 78. The cultural and microscopic characteristics of *Rhizopus* species

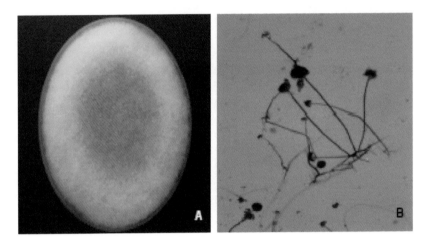

Basidiobolus species

- Colonies are moderately fast-growing at 30°C, flat, creamy-grey, radially folded and covered by a fine, powdery, white aerial mycelium (Fig. 79A).
- Satellite colonies are often formed by germinating conidia ejected from the primary colony.
- Large vegetative hyphae, thick-walled zygospores with two closely appressed beak-like appendages (Fig. 79B, C).

Figure 79. The cultural and microscopic characteristics of *Basidiobolus* species

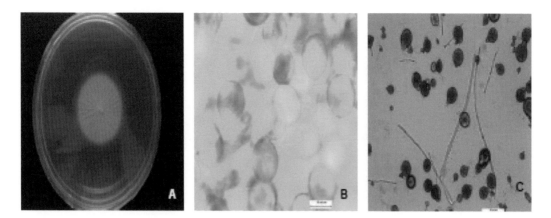

Syncephalastrum species

- Colonies grow rapidly and are cottony or woolly due to abundant aerial mycelium. Initially white becoming dark grey (Fig. 80A).
- Hyphae are hyaline, broad, and non-septated.
- Sporangiophores are short; branches arise from rhizoids, the end of each branch enlarges to form a vesicle.
- On the vesicle are merosporangia, each containing a linear chain of about 18 merospores (merosporangiospores) (Fig. 80B).
- Merosporangiospores are single-celled, spherical in shape.

Figure 80. The cultural and microscopic characteristics of *Syncephalastrum species*

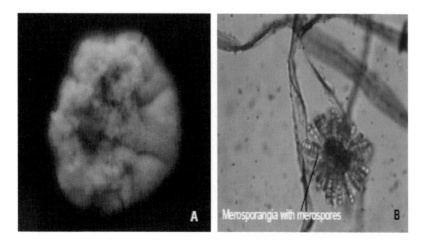

Cunninghamella species

- Colonies grow rapidly and are floccose with tuffs of short aerial mycelium. Colonies are initially white and then become tannish-grey (Fig. 81A).
- Hyphae are hyaline, broad, and non-septated.
- Sporangiophores are long, with whorls of short lateral branches; each branch terminates in a swollen vesicle.

- Each vesicle has spine-like denticles covering the entire surface; attached to each denticle are round-oval sporangioles with one sporangiospore (Fig. 81B).
- Sporangiospores are one-celled and globose to ovoid in shape.

Figure 81. The cultural and microscopic characteristics of *Cunninghamella* species

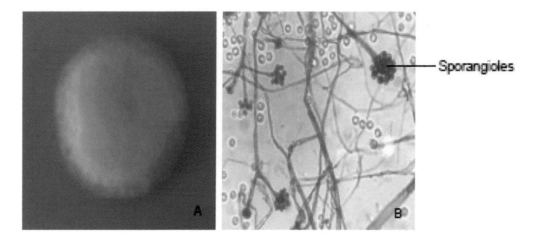

Section 7. Dimorphic Fungi

Fungi can exist in moulds, filamentous, or yeast forms depending on the growth temperatures. At 37°C or in tissues, the fungus exists in yeast form; at room temperature or 30°C the fungus exists in mould form.

Three examples of dimorphic fungi: *Histoplasma capsulatum, Sporothrix schenckii* and *Penicillium marneffei.*

Histoplasma capsulatum

- Colonies grow slowly and are compact or velvety with a button-like central elevation. Initially white or tan becoming brownish with white compacted mycelium.
- Hyphae are hyaline, septate with short conidiophores bearing a characteristic large, rounded, tuberculated macroconidia (Fig. 82A).
- Microconidia are small, rounded, located on short conidiophores branching directly from the sides of the hyphae.
- Thermo-dimorphism can be demonstrated by inoculating the fungus on enriched medium e.g. brain-heart-infusion-blood agar incubated at 37°C with the production of white and smooth yeast-like colonies.
- In infected tissue, the organism appears as yeast-like cells with budding; the cell wall stains intensely with a thin clear space or halo around the cells (Fig. 82B).
- A *Histoplasma* isolate that shows no thermal dimorphism is a *Sepedonium* species (Fig. 62).

Figure 82. Direct microscopic examination of *Histoplasma capsulatum* in blood culture (A) and tissue (B)

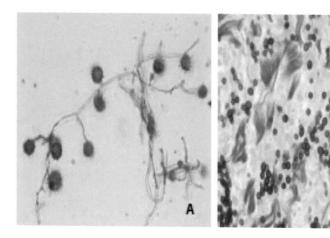

Penicillium marneffei

- At room temperature (30°C), colonies grow moderately rapidly and are velvety with raised centers, producing a distinctive pink pigment that diffuses into the medium (Fig. 83A).
- Hyphae are septate, penicilli biverticillate with long smooth conidiophores (Fig. 83B).
- At 37°C on enriched medium, colonies are yeast-like, small, rough and white in colour (Fig. 83C).
- Gram stain shows ellipsoidal to spherical yeast-like cells and long pseudomycelium (Fig. 83D).

Figure 83. Thermo-dimorphism of *Penicillium marneffei* demonstrated by different incubating temperatures

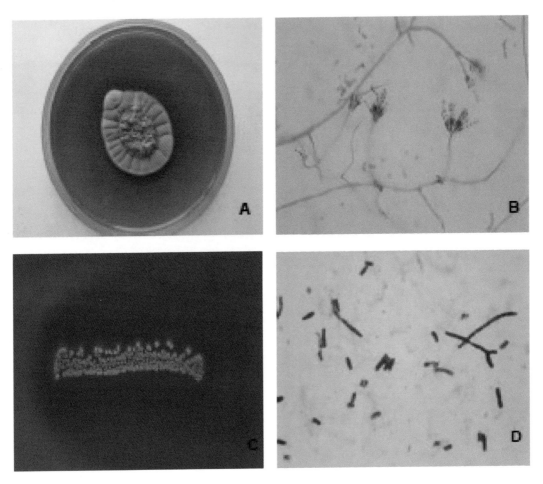

Sporothrix schenckii

- At room temperature (30°C), colonies are slow-growing, with a folded and wrinkled surface, light grey to black (Fig. 84A).
- Conidiophores are erect, short, and thin, usually single arising from the septated hyphae. Conidia are in clusters or single with tiny denticles proliferating at the apex of the conidiophores (Fig. 84B).
- On blood agar incubated at 37°C, colonies are yeast-like, with punctuated center, white in colour (Fig. 84C).

68

- Gram stain shows spherical or oval budding yeast cells with pseudohyphae (Fig. 84D).

Figure 84. Thermo-dimorphism of *Sporothrix schenckii* demonstrated by different incubating temperatures

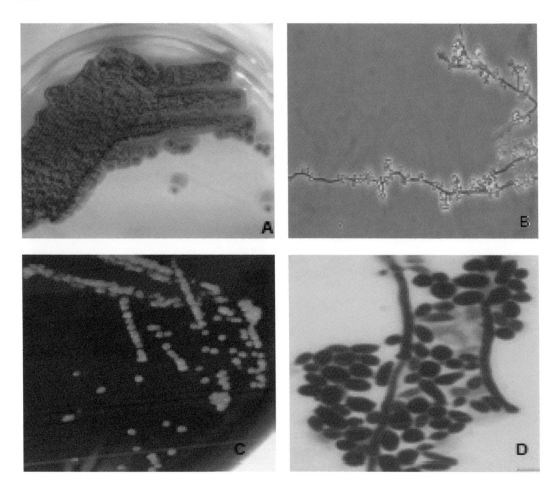

Section 8. Dematiaceous Hyphomycetes

Dematiaceous Hyphomycetes are conidial fungi that produce dark brown, green-black, or black colonies; they are the causative agents of chromomycosis and phaeohyphomycosis.

Alternaria species

- Colonies grow rapidly and are flat and olivaceous-black. The reverse side is typically black.
- Hyphae and conidiophores are septate.
- Microscopically, branched acropetal chains of multi-celled conidia are produced from conidiophores.
- Conidia are brown, smooth-walled or verrucose with longitudinal and transverse septations, single or catenate, round base with a short pointed apex (Fig. 85).
- About 50 species, most commonly isolated human pathogen: *Alternaria alternata*, *Alternaria tenuissima.*

Figure 85. The typical chains of multi-celled conidia of *Alternaria* species

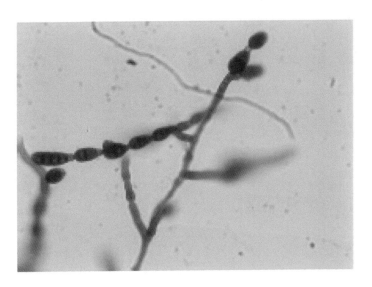

Alternaria alternata

- Colonies grow rapidly and are grey to olivaceous black, felty with dense aerial mycelium (Fig. 86A).
- Conidiophores are unbranched, conidia obclavate with muriform septation and a short cylindrical beak at the base. Conidia in chain of ten or more with a single scar at the tip (Fig. 86B).

Figure 86. The cultural and microscopic characteristics of *Alternaria alternata*

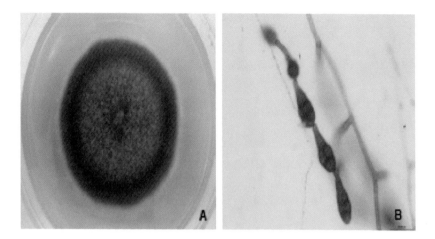

Curvularia species

- Colonies are fast growing, woolly, velvety to floccose, and blackish brown. The reverse is black.
- Conidiophore is erect, single, or branched, and geniculate where conidium forms.
- Conidia cluster at the tip of conidiophores.
- The transverse septa divide each conidium into four cells; the conidium is slightly curved because the central cell is larger and darker than others (Fig. 87).
- The identification of the species is based on the characteristic appearance of the conidium.

Figure 87. The microscopic characteristics of *Curvularia* species

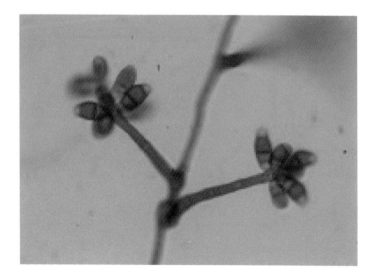

Curvularia lunata

- Colonies grow rapidly and are black, expanding, and floccose with radial, deep fissures (Fig. 88A).
- Conidiophores are septate, erect and unbranched, geniculate with conidia in sympodial patterns.
- Conidia are smooth-walled, three-septa, obovoidal, curved with subterminal cell larger than the others (Fig. 88B).

Figure 88. The cultural and microscopic characteristics of *Curvularia lunata*

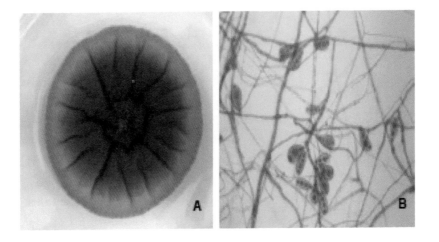

Curvularia clavata

- Colonies grow rapidly and are initially white becoming greyish-brown, spreading, floccose or cottony with tuffs of aerial mycelium (Fig. 89A).
- Conidiophores are erect, single, unbranched, long, and geniculate; the cluster of conidia is at the tip of conidiophores (Fig. 89B).
- Conidia are fusiform, smooth-walled, and slightly curved with three transverse septa.

Figure 89. The cultural and microscopic characteristics of *Curvularia clavata*

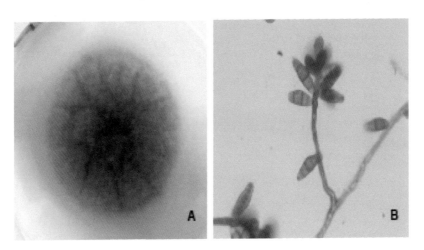

Fonsecaea species

- Colonies grow slowly and are compact, slightly raised, velvety, olivaceous to brown-black in both front and the reverse (Fig. 90A).
- Hyphae are septate, branched, and dark brown in colour. The conidiogenous cell is always confined to the tip of the conidiophores.
- The fungus is identified by the presence of four types of conidium production: cladosporium type, sympodial type, fonsecaea type and phialophora type (Fig. 90B, C)

Figure 90. The cultural and microscopic characteristics of *Fonsecaea* species

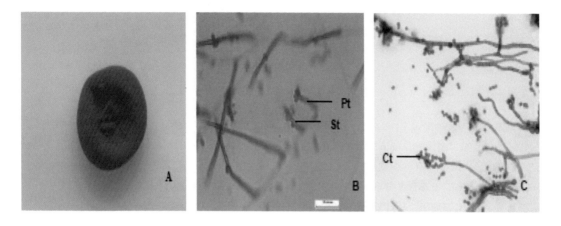

Pt : phialophora type   Ct : cladosporium type   St : sympodial type

Bipolaris species

- Colonies are fast growing and compact with abundant short aerial mycelium, and olivaceous black with a black reverse (Fig. 91A).
- Conidiophores are simple or branched, flexuose with zigzag rachis bearing conidium in a sympodial pattern (Fig. 91B).
- Conidia are distoseptate, usually four cells, fusiform to ellipsoidal, and rounded at both ends.
- Important species: *Bipolaris australiensis*, *Bipolaris hawaiiensis* and *Bipolaris spicifera*.

Figure 91. The cultural and microscopic characteristics of *Bipolaris species*

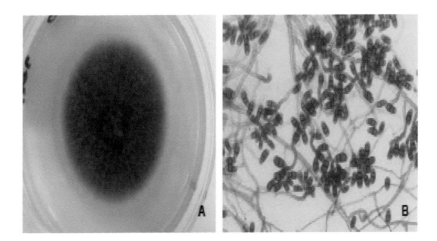

Hortaea werneckii

- Colonies grow rapidly and are olivaceous black both in front and on the reverse (Fig. 92A).
- Exhibit both a yeast-like and hyphal morphology.
- Yeast cells with thick septum; the budding may be polar, bipolar, or lateral (Fig. 92B).
- On Gomori methanamine silver nitrate stain (GMS), the surface of some of the yeast cells is marked by conspicuous rings or collarette intercalary or laterally (Fig. 93).
- Halophilic black yeast grows abundantly in 10% Nacl incubated at room temperature.

Figure 92. The cultural and microscopic characteristics of *Hortaea werneckii*

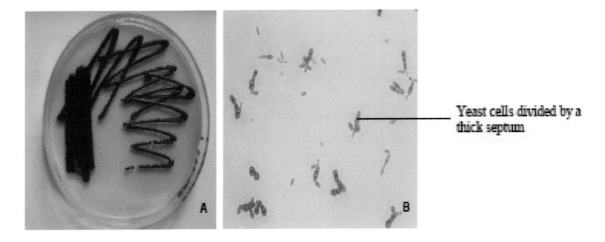

Yeast cells divided by a thick septum

Figure 93. Gomori methanamine silver nitrate stain; note melanin, collarette and red stained nuclei (x100)

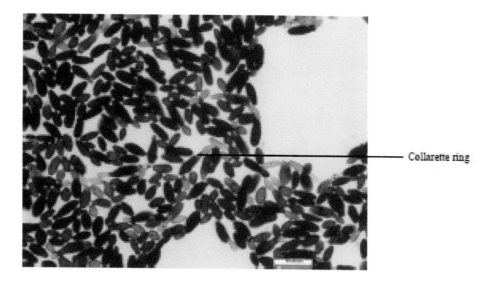

Collarette ring

Exophiala species

- Colonies are initially yeast-like, moist, slimy at the center, and smooth near the margin; later they become velvety due to dense aerial mycelium, olivaceous-black (Fig. 94A).
- Yeast cells are predominant in young culture; septate hyphae bear intercalary, cylindrical, or flask-shaped conidiogenous cells with single or several short annellated zones (Fig. 94B, C).
- Conidia are ellipsoidal, usually one-celled in clusters at the apices of conidiogenous cells.

Figure 94. The cultural and microscopic characteristics of *Exophiala* species

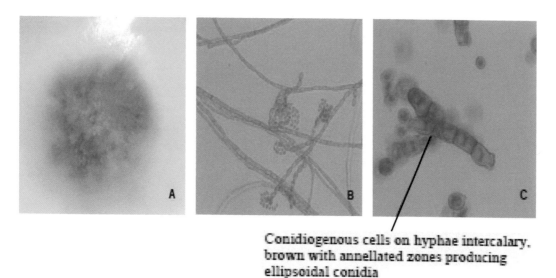

Conidiogenous cells on hyphae intercalary, brown with annellated zones producing ellipsoidal conidia

Cladosporium species

- Colonies grow rapidly and are velvety to powdery, olivaceous black. The reverse of the colony is black (Fig. 95A).

- Hyphae are dark and segmented. Conidiophores variable in length, branched or unbranched, nodose, or geniculate. The ramoconidia frequently observed (Fig. 95B).
- Conidiogenous cells (ramoconidia) with lateral ramifications produce chains of conidia.
- Ramoconidium is usually followed by a septate secondary ramoconidium, smaller intercalary conidia, and very small usually aseptate terminal conidia (Fig. 95C).

Figure 95. The cultural and microscopic characteristics of *Cladosporium* species

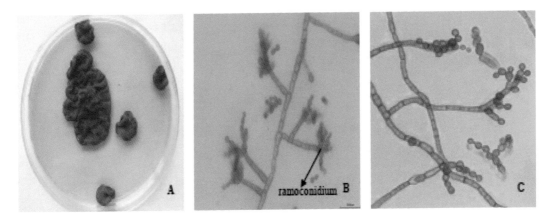

Cladosporium oxysporum

- Colonies grow moderately and are olivaceous green, velvety or floccose (Fig. 96A).
- Conidiophores are unbranched, septate, straight, or flexuous with terminal or lateral ramifications bearing chains of conidia (Fig. 96B).
- Ramoconidia cylindrical to clavate, 0-1 septate with obvious scar.
- Terminal conidia are ellipsoidal or subglobose; wall is smooth.

Figure 96. The cultural and microscopic characteristics of *Cladosporium oxysporum*

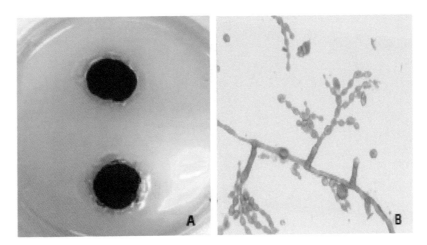

Cladosporium sphaerospermum

- Colonies grow moderately rapid and are olivaceous brown, velvety, and furrowed with a wrinkled center (Fig. 97A). Reverse is black in colour.

- Conidiophores are variable in length, not geniculate, smooth-walled, and branched with thick septa (Fig. 97B).
- Produce ramoconidia, 0-3 septate, elongated and smooth-walled.
- Terminal aseptate conidia are globose to subglobose, brown to dark brown in colour with prominent a scar (Fig. 97C).

Figure 97. The cultural and microscopic characteristics of *Cladosporium sphaerospermum*

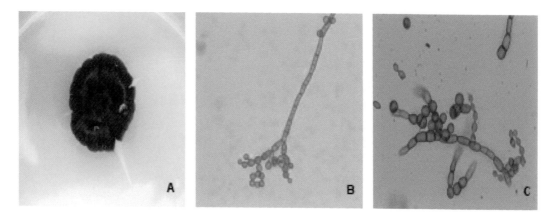

Hendersonula toruloidea

- Colonies grow rapidly and are woolly with tuffs of aerial mycelium, initially white becoming olivaceous black later (Fig. 98A). Reverse is black.
- Hyphae are septate, and break up into long chains of arthroconidia (Fig. 98B).
- Arthroconidia may be square or oval.

Figure 98. The cultural and microscopic characteristics of *Hendersonula toruloidea*

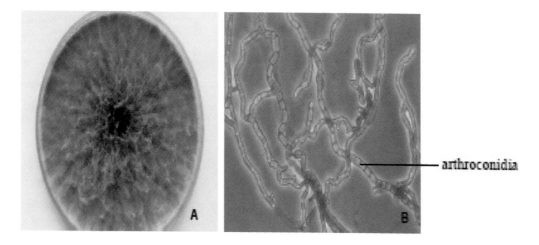

Exserohilum species

- Colonies grow rapidly and are woolly, dark grey to brownish-black with a black reverse (Fig. 99A).
- Septate hyphae. Conidiophores simple, long, septate, and appear as zigzag form or geniculate where they bend at the points of formation of conidia.

- Conidia are fusiform, straight to slightly curved with 3-12 pseudoseptate (Fig. 99B).
- A protuberant hilum is present at the base; the septum of the terminal cells is thickened.
- Important species: *Exserohilum rostratum,* the conidia slightly curved, 3-9 pseudoseptate with thickened septum at both ends.

Figure 99. The cultural and microscopic characteristics of *Exserohilum* species

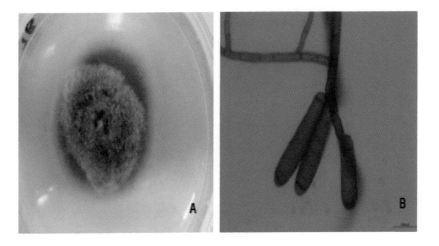

Phialophora species

- Colonies grow slowly and are woolly to velvety, olivaecous black with the reverse side grey to black (Fig. 100A).
- Hyphae are septate; the conidiophores have short phialides. The phialides could be flask or cylindrical shaped depending on the species.
- Conidia are unicellular, brown, oval, and accumulate as masses at the apices of phialides (Fig. 100B).

Figure 100. The cultural and microscopic characteristics of *Phialophora* species

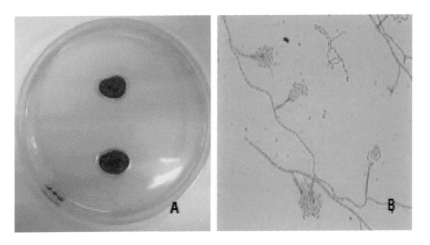

Nigrospora species

- Colonies grow rapidly and are cottony, initially white, and become black when sporulation is abundant (Fig. 101A).
- Hyphae are septate; conidiophore short producing swollen and ampulliform conidiogenous cells.
- Conidiogenous cells bear a large, single, unicellular conidium.
- Conidia are spherical, solitary, black, slightly flattened horizontally with an equatorial slit (Fig. 101B).
- Important species: *Nigrospora sphaerica*.

Figure 101. The cultural and microscopic characteristics of *Nigrospora* species

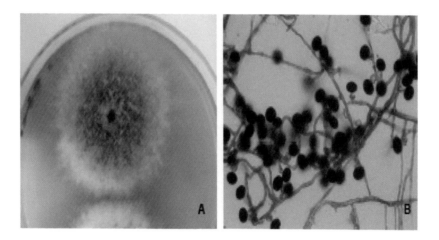

Ochroconis species

- An emerging human opportunistic pathogen especially in transplant recipients.
- Colonies grow rapidly, some strains produce diffusible pigments.

Ochroconis constricta

- Colonies grow slowly and are restricted with tuffs of short aerial mycelium centrally, greyish-brown with dark brown diffusible pigment at the periphery (Fig. 102A).
- Hyphae are septate, smooth to rough-walled.
- Conidiophores are poorly differentiated, arising from the side of hyphae, cylindrical bearing 3-6 conidia on denticles at the tip (Fig. 102B).
- Conidia are two-celled, rough-walled, and ellipsoidal with rounded ends.

Figure 102. The cultural and microscopic characteristics of *Ochroconis constricta*

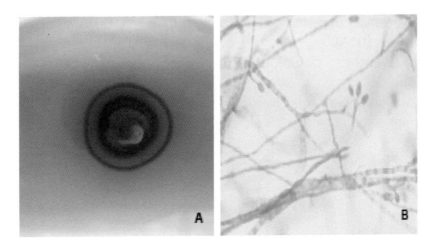

Ochroconis gallopava

- Colonies grow slowly and are floccose with tuffs of aerial mycelium centrally, olivaceous-brown with dark-brown pigments diffused into the media (Fig. 103A).
- Conidiophores poorly differentiated, nearing a single conidium at the tip (Fig. 103B).
- Conidia are two-celled and smooth-walled; the apical cell is wider than the basal cell.

Figure 103. The cultural and microscopic characteristics of *Ochroconis gallopava*

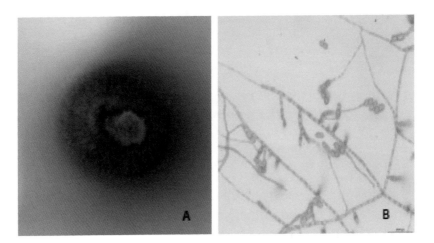

Phoma species

- Colonies grow slowly and are fluffy with prominent radial folds; pale to grey (Fig. 104A).
- Produce dark coloured pycnidia with single ostiole or multi-ostiolate. The pycnidia may be single or aggregated in groups (Fig. 104B).
- Conidiogenous cells lined on the inner wall of pycnidium; conidia mostly unicellular, pale, ellipsoidal, fusiform or other forms; may have a septum (Fig. 104C).
- Chlamydospores arrange in chains, with oblique, longitudinal and transverse septa (Fig. 104D).

Figure 104. The cultural and microscopic characteristics of *Phoma* species

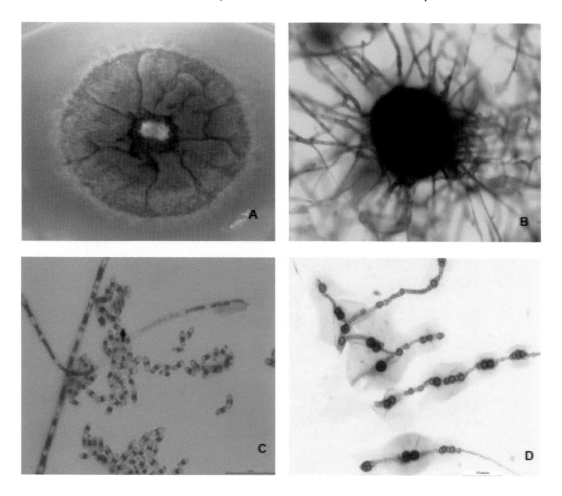

Chaetomium species

- Colonies grow and expand rapidly and are abundant white or grey aerial mycelium (Fig. 105A).
- Perithecium (ascomata/fruiting body) is subspherical to pyriform; single ostiole with unbranched ascomatal setae covers the entire surface (Fig. 105B).
- They usually produce 4-8 ascospores: cylindrical, obovoidal, or fusiform.

Figure 105. The cultural and microscopic characteristics of *Chaetomium* species

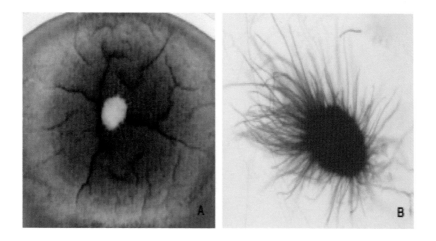

Daldinia species

- Colonies grow rapidly and are felty or cottony with tuffs of aerial mycelium; whitish in colour (Fig. 106A).
- Hyphae are septate; conidiophores branch irregularly with conidiogenous cells arising from the terminus (Fig. 106B).
- Conidia are ellipsoid in shape; cluster at the tip of a short, poorly differentiated conidiophores.

Figure 106. The cultural and microscopic characteristics of *Daldinia* species

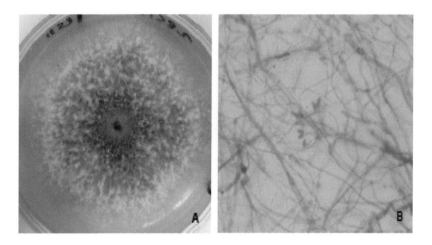

Section 9. Non-cultivable Fungus

Pneumocystis species

- In the family Pneumocystidaceae, there is only one medically important species: *Pneumocystis jirovecii (Pneumocystis carinii)*, a yeast-like fungus.
- The fungus cannot be cultured on laboratory medium.
- The infection can only be diagnosed by Giemsa stain, Grocott methenamine silver nitrate stain (GMS), immunofluorescent stain, or PCR. The specimens frequently used are bronchioalveolar lavage or induced sputum specimens.
- On biopsied lung tissue, non-budding yeast cells, cup-shaped or crescent-shaped cysts measuring 4-8 μm are the diagnostic features (Fig. 107).

Figure 107. *Pneumocystis jirovecii* in tissue

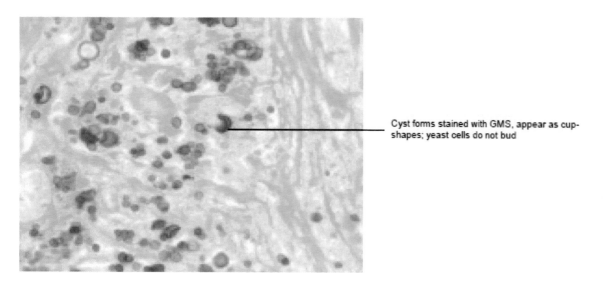

Cyst forms stained with GMS, appear as cup-shapes; yeast cells do not bud

Bibliography

1. Chandler, F.W., Kaplan, W. & Ajello, L., 1980. A Colour Atlas of the Histopathology of Mycotic Diseases. Wolfe Medical Publications Ltd., London.
2. De Hoog, G.S., Guarro, J., Gene, J. & Figueras, M.J., 2nd edition, 2000. Atlas of Clinical Fungi. Centraalbureau voor Schimmelcultures, Utrecht, The Netherlands.
3. Delacretaz, J., Grigoriu, D. & Ducel, G., 1974. Color Atlas of Medical Mycology. Hans Huber Publishers, Bern Stuttgart, Vienna.
4. Ellis, D., Davis, S., Alexiou, H., Handke, R. & Bartley, R., 2007. Descriptions of Medical Fungi. 2nd Edition. Nexus Print Solutions, Underdale, South Australia.
5. Ellis, M.B., 1971. Dematiaceous Hyphomycetes. Commonwealth Mycological Institute, Kew, Surrey, England.
6. Kreger-van Rij, N.J.W. (ed.), 1984. The Yeasts a Taxonomic Study. Elsevier Science Publishers, BV Amsterdam.
7. Larone. D.H., 3rd Edition, 1995. Medically Important Fungi: a guide to identification. American Society for Microbiology, Washington.
8. McGinnis, M.R., 1980. Laboratory Handbook of Medical Mycology. Academic Press Inc, New York and London.
9. Mycology online. www.**mycology**.adelaide.edu.au
10. Ramirez, C. & Martinez, A.T., 1982. Manual and Atlas of the Penicillia. Elsevier Biomedical Press, Amsterdam, New York and Oxford.
11. Samson, R.A. & Pitt, J.I., (ed.), 2000. Integration of Modern Taxonomic Methods for *Penicillium* and *Aspergillus* Classification. Harwood Academic Publishers, Australia.